CURRENT ISSUES IN CANCER

CURRENT ISSUES IN CANCER

Published by the BMJ Publishing Group
Tavistock Square, London WC1H 9JR

First published 1992

British Library Cataloguing in Publication Data
A catalogue record for this book is available from the British Library

ISBN 0 7279 0775 1

The following picture sources are acknowledged:

Page 81, P Marazzi, Science Photo Library; page 82, St Bartholomew's Medical Illustration Department; page 127, St James's University; page 137, M Wilson, Format.

Typeset by Bedford Typesetters Limited, Bedford
Printed and bound in Great Britain by
Latimer Trend & Company Ltd, Plymouth

Contents

CURRENT ISSUES IN CANCER

Introduction

The past 50 years have seen an enormous proliferation of interest in the causes and treatment of cancer. The diminishing threat of death from infectious diseases and the increasing longevity of populations throughout the world have highlighted the importance of cancers, many of which continue to increase in incidence.

This series of articles, originally published in the *British Medical Journal*, examines the present state of management of a number of malignancies, and also attempts to increase understanding of the biology of these diseases, their treatments, and their impact on people.

There have been great strides in our understanding of the genetic mechanisms underlying cancer. Known hereditary cancer syndromes have been matched with abnormalities at the genetic level; oncogenes in certain cancer types have been recognised and described, opening a window to the underlying genetic events and to future possible therapeutic targets.

Though, perhaps inevitably, the treatment of cancer has lagged behind such scientific discoveries, we are increasingly using our knowledge of the biology of tumours in their management. In particular our new understanding of histogenesis in lymphoma has been used in classification and has been related to differences in clinical behaviour, response to treatment, and outcome. Similarly, in early stage breast cancer appropriate use of adjuvant treatment now extends far beyond consideration of the stage alone and is increasingly related to the biological features of the disease. Of course, of equal importance, our increased awareness of how early breast cancer spreads has enabled previously routine mutilating operations to become a thing of the past.

The outstanding success of the past 20 years has been in the management of testicular cancer. Perhaps typically, most of the advances have been based on the empirical introduction of different chemotherapeutic drugs, in particular cisplatin. The therapeutic yield has been great, and the structured research approach has provided a model for work on other cancers. By contrast colorectal cancer has been something of a cinderella within oncology. Even in this area, however, adjuvant treatments seem to be yielding a survival advantage in selected subgroups, and an increasing awareness of the importance of surgical specialisation (and perhaps, in the future, screening) should bring about significant benefits. Lung cancer remains an almost overwhelming international problem. Here, too, the biology is now better defined, and while therapeutic advances have been slow, there has been more integration of surgery, radiotherapy, and chemotherapy, and better recognition of cases appropriate for radical versus palliative treatment approaches.

What about therapeutic advances for the future? Improvements in radiotherapy are taking place at present—both by increasing the therapeutic index and also by more accurate, and thereby less damaging, treatment of tumour bearing areas. Biological therapy offers an entirely different approach to the management of cancer, and several authors have suggested that the rather crude treatments available today put us in a situation similar to that when the first alkylating agents were introduced in the mid-1940s. It seems likely that the increasing definition of malignancy will allow "tailored" biological therapy to be produced in the future, which may interact specifically with cancer cells, or alternatively influence the mechanisms underlying cell division.

Despite the excitement caused by current therapeutic advances we cannot forget the impact of cancer and its treatment on our patients. Quality of life in all its senses has become an increasingly important issue and is now routinely evaluated in many cancer trials.

This volume does not aim to be comprehensive, nor is it intended to act as a text book. We hope, however, that it provides a refreshing look at the present state of knowledge and treatment in the cancers included, as well as a glimpse of the future.

G M MEAD

Molecular genetics of cancer

B A J PONDER

Cancer as a genetic disease

Several steps are needed to turn a normal cell into a cancer cell. Most, if not all, of these include mutational change. Cancer is therefore a genetic disease at the level of the cell. It may also be a genetic disease at the level of inheritance. Many of the "cancer genes" have important normal functions in the control of growth and development. The rapidly growing understanding of the genetics of cancer is leading in two directions—towards new approaches to treatment and prevention and towards a deeper insight into the central problems of cell biology.

Accumulation of mutations in a cell

Most cancers start from a single cell. This cell and its descendants must have accumulated mutations in several different genes before they become cancer.[1] Some of the later stages of this accumulation may be reflected in abnormal behaviour of the cell and be recognised by the pathologist as increasing degrees of premalignant change, such as dysplasia. However, we have not yet generally reached the point where specific pathological features can be related to mutation in specific genes.

Mutations in tissue cells accumulate continually throughout life, beginning in the embryo. As we grow older, each of us is an increasingly complex mosaic of mutant cells and their progeny. Whether in any one of us a complete set of critical mutations coincides within the same cell and leads to cancer depends, no doubt, on luck; but it also depends on the environmental, behavioural, and inherited

1

factors that determine whether our cells are exposed to potential mutagens and how we deal with the consequences. In other words, cancer risk depends not only on environmental exposure but also on genetic make up. In a few people the inherited factor is particularly strong. In the race to accumulate mutations, these people have a head start because they have already inherited a critical mutation in every cell, through the germline. They, and their family members who have inherited the same mutation, are much more likely to develop cancer and may be recognisable as part of a "cancer family."[2]

Critical genes

Most cancer genes that have been identified so far belong to one or another of the chains of command within the cell for the control of growth or differentiation (table I). Conceptually, they fall into two groups: oncogenes,[3 4] mutations of which lead to altered activity or increased expression of the corresponding protein, which has a positive effect in driving the cell towards malignancy, and suppressor genes,[5] mutations of which result in loss of activity or expression of the corresponding protein, and thereby loss of a normal function of regulation or restraint. Not surprisingly, the types of mutation which activate oncogenes or lose activity of suppressor genes tend to be different.

Oncogenes

Oncogenes may be activated by a change in a single amino acid, leading, for example, to an altered shape of the protein; by multiplication of the gene within the chromosome to provide several copies

TABLE I—Examples of oncogenes and suppressor genes and their role in pathways of cellular growth control*

Soluble growth factors	sis
Cell surface growth factor receptor	erb B, fms, neu
Transduction of signals within the cell	ras family, src abl
Nuclear proteins concerned with DNA replication and gene transcription	myc, fos, myb Rb, Wilms, p53

*Growth control molecules outside the cell act by binding to cell surface receptors. The signals are relayed from the inner surface of these receptors across the cytoplasm to the nucleus, where they affect DNA replication or gene expression. Many of the genes which are mutated in cancer cells or which are implicated in inherited predisposition to cancer lie at one point or another on these control pathways.

and thus increased activity (amplification); or by rearrangements of genes between chromosomes so that functional regions of the oncogene are brought under different and inappropriate control. The first oncogenes were identified by experiments in which DNA from cancer cells was broken into small pieces and introduced into mouse fibroblasts in culture. The presence of activated oncogenes caused the mouse cells that received them to grow abnormally, and it was fairly straightforward to isolate these "transformed" cells and identify the human DNA sequences within them that were responsible. Subsequently, other oncogenes have been identified by their presence at the points of critical chromosome rearrangements in cancers—for example, the abl gene, which is activated by the chromosome 9-22 rearrangement in chronic myeloid leukaemia.

Suppressor genes

Suppressor genes are more difficult to find because it is much more difficult to set up an assay to look for a negative activity. The existence of suppressor genes was predicted over 20 years ago by Knudson.[6] Figure 1 shows the hypothesis he proposed to account for the observation that hereditary and sporadic cases of retinoblastoma are histologically and clinically indistinguishable but that the hereditary cases occur on average earlier and are often multiple. The hypothesis

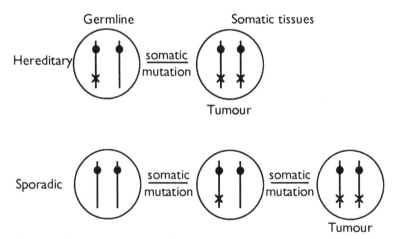

Figure 1—Knudson's hypothesis. The two chromosomes of a pair are shown with mutation (X) at the locus of a cancer gene. Whereas only one further (somatic) mutation is required for tumour formation in hereditary cases, two mutations within the same cell are required in sporadic cases

3

states that both copies of a critical gene must be lost from a cell for a tumour to develop. In hereditary cases one loss is inherited as a mutation in the germline and is therefore already present in every cell in the target tissue. In this case, the chances are very high that loss of the second copy will subsequently occur by mutation in at least one cell of the tissue, and one or several tumours will almost certainly result. In sporadic cases, by contrast, both mutations have to occur by chance as somatic mutations in the same cell. This coincidence will be rare, so sporadic tumours will be uncommon (in retinoblastoma, about 1 in 100 000 children) and on average they will take longer to occur; multiple tumours in the same child will be so unlikely as to be almost diagnostic of an inherited predisposition. Ten years after this hypothesis the germline retinoblastoma (Rb) mutation was located on chromosome 13, and shortly after that Knudson's hypothesis was confirmed by the finding that in retinoblastoma tumours both copies of the Rb gene were indeed inactivated by mutation.[7] A similar genetic mechanism probably underlies the other inherited cancer syndromes such as familial polyposis of the colon, multiple endocrine neoplasia, and neurofibromatosis.

Although the idea of suppressor genes was developed from studies of inherited cancers, their importance is not confined to these cases.

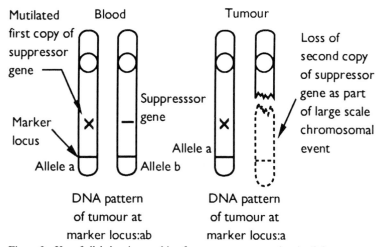

DNA pattern of tumour at marker locus:ab   DNA pattern of tumour at marker locus:a

Figure 2—Use of allele loss in searching for suppressor genes. A pair of chromosomes which carry a locus for a suppressor gene is shown. Loss of the second copy of the suppressor gene is accompanied by large scale loss of chromosomal material from that region, which is detected as loss of one allele (b) at a marker locus on the chromosome

The role of suppressor gene mutations in sporadic cancers has been shown by studies of so called "allele loss" or "loss of heterozygosity" (fig 2). The principle is straightforward. The mutational event which results in loss of the second copy of the gene is often accompanied by a large scale chromosomal rearrangement or deletion. Because it is a large scale event, this is relatively easy to detect by using sets of DNA markers which have two alleles, each allele being present in one of the chromosomes of a pair. DNA from the tumour is compared with DNA from the patient's blood. The consistent loss of one allele of the pair in a particular chromosomal region in the tumour DNA strongly suggests that loss of genes from this region is a necessary feature of tumour development, and it implies the presence in that region of one or more suppressor genes (table II). Many laboratories worldwide are now trying to identify the specific genes involved.

Like the Rb gene, some of these genes may be the targets of inherited mutations in the inherited cancer syndromes, as well as having a role in the development of sporadic tumours. Thus, the detailed analysis of allele losses in common colon cancers pinpointed the location of the familial polyposis gene on chromosome 5, and a similar strategy is being used to find the other genes responsible for inherited breast and ovarian cancer. Other suppressor genes seem to act only through somatic mutations as part of tumour development, perhaps because these mutations would be lethal to the development of the embryo if they were inherited.

TABLE II—Chromosomal locations of probable tumour suppressor genes acting in some common cancers

Cancer	Chromosomal region (p=short arm, q=long arm)
Breast	1p 1q 3p 6q 11p 13q 16q 17p 17q 18 22
Colorectal	1p 5q 17p 18q 22
Small cell lung cancer	3p 11p 13q 17p
Glioma	9p 10 17p 22q
Prostate	8p 10q 16q
Renal	3p 5q 10 13q 18

Note that some regions are often involved, which suggests that losses of some suppressor genes may be common to the development of many different cancers. However, some chromosome regions (for example, 3p, 17p, 17q) probably contain several different suppressor gene loci.

5

> ## Features that may suggest the presence of inherited predisposition
>
> 1 Uncommon cancers in two or more close blood relatives
> 2 Common cancer at a young age (<45 years) in close blood relatives
> 3 Bilateral or multiple primary cancers
> 4 Associated non-cancerous abnormalities:
>   Developmental abnormalities (see table III)
>   Marker phenotypes—colon cancer with multiple polyps, melanoma with atypical naevi

Inherited predisposition to cancer

Perhaps 5-10% of common cancers (breast, ovarian, colonic) occur in familial clusters which are the result of genetic susceptibility.[8 9] Relatives in some of these families may have lifetime risks of specific cancers as high as 30-40%. The problem, of course, is that cancer is a common disease and so some family clusters may be simply due to chance. Because of this, family histories are often ignored. If there is a very strong family history, as in the example in figure 3, genetic predisposition is in little doubt. Less striking family histories may be more difficult to identify, and the box lists some family histories that are likely to be important. A characteristic phenotype caused by the inherited gene mutation provides unambiguous recognition of some of the inherited cancer syndromes (table III), and should be searched for even in isolated cases of these tumours in young people. The clinical implications will be discussed below.

Predisposition in these families is usually due to a single dominantly inherited gene, which means that the child of an affected parent is at 50% risk of inheriting the predisposition. However, the chances that the gene will result in cancer may vary both within and between families and will be related to age, so that the risk to an individual will usually be spread over many years and some carriers of the gene may never develop the cancer at all. In multiple case families, it is possible to search for the predisposing genes by genetic linkage.[10] The inheritance of a series of marker genes through the family is studied until a marker is found, the inheritance of which coincides with that of the cancer. The cancer gene and the marker gene must lie close together on a chromosome, otherwise their inheritance would become

6

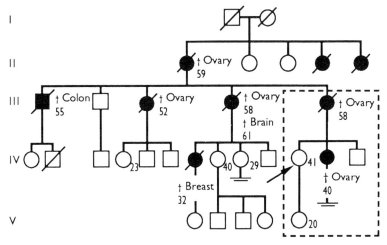

Figure 3—Pedigree of family with ovarian, breast, and colon cancer. The 41 year old woman (arrowed) in generation IV sought advice. Her history was of an affected sister and mother (dotted rectangle), which is suggestive of predisposition. Further investigation of family history provided stronger evidence and indicated other family members at risk (indicated by age)

separated by genetic crossing over in each generation. The recent rapid development of the human gene map has provided many hundreds of gene markers, and as a result many of the genes for the more striking familial cancers have already been located (table IV). To move from this mapping of a gene to the isolation of the gene itself is a laborious process, but five such genes have now been found, each of

TABLE III—Examples of associated abnormalities in inherited cancer syndromes

Syndrome	Tissues principally affected by tumour	Characteristic associated abnormalities
Familial adenomatous polyposis	Colon (small intestine, thyroid, liver)	Multiple colonic polyps, hypertrophy of retinal pigment epithelium, desmoid tumours
Von Hippel-Lindau disease	Kidney, adrenal medulla, haemangioblastoma of cerebellum	Angiomas of retina, multiple cysts of internal organs
Neurofibromatosis type 1	Glia, adrenal medulla, Schwann cells	Multiple: including café au lait spots, cutaneous neurofibroma, scoliosis, axillary freckling, short stature
Dysplastic naevus syndrome	Melanoma	Atypical (large, irregular, unusually pigmented) naevi

7

TABLE IV—Localisation of some inherited genes predisposing to cancer

Cancer	Chromosome
Colon (familial adenomatous polyposis)	5q
Breast (also families with breast and ovarian cancer)	17q
Pituitary, adrenal, pancreatic islets (multiple endocrine neoplasia type I)	11q
Thyroid C cell, phaeochromocytoma (multiple endocrine neoplasia type II)	10
Kidney (von Hippel-Lindau disease)	3p
Glioma (neurofibromatosis type 1)	17q
Retina, bone (retinoblastoma, osteosarcoma)	13q

which seems to have a normal function in some aspect of the control of cell proliferation or differentiation. More will certainly follow.

Progress has been made with the clear cut inherited cancer syndromes such as familial polyposis because the genetic predisposition is strong and therefore relatively well defined and easy to analyse. It is important to realise, however, that in cancer (as in other common diseases with an inherited component, such as atherosclerotic heart disease) such extreme effects account for only a small part of the population burden of the disease. There are almost certainly many commoner predisposing genes which have weaker effects, so that even in a gene carrier the risk of the specific cancer may be only (say) 10%. These genes will be hard to spot because there will be hardly any familial clustering: most people in the family who have inherited the gene will not have cancer. Even so, it is easy to show that at the population level the genes could result in most of the cases of a specific cancer occurring within a predisposed minority of the population.[8] If true, this has obvious implications for screening and prevention. Interactions between genes and the environment may also be important. Evidence is already emerging, for example, that the risk of lung cancer from cigarette smoking is higher in a genetically predisposed group within the population.[11] Because genetic predisposition is likely to affect many more people than the clear cut family cancer syndromes, in the long term it may be of much greater importance for public health.

Clinical implications

Inherited predisposition

Some familial cancers offer the opportunity to identify people at high risk to enable screening or prevention. For example, families with the dysplastic naevus syndrome may be at very high risk of melanoma.[12] They should protect their children from sunburn, and from puberty onwards family members should have regular checks and excision of suspicious naevi. An apparently isolated case of haemangioblastoma of the cerebellum may have occurred in someone coming from a family with von Hippel-Lindau disease. Such families are at risk of kidney cancer in middle age and will probably benefit from screening.[13] These conditions are uncommon, but if family histories are not taken opportunities will be lost. The families themselves are usually already aware that something is amiss and will welcome advice. Of course, there are difficult cases. The significance of the family history may not be clear (is the occurrence of breast cancer in two sisters at age 45 important?) or it may not be clear who will benefit from genetic advice (is breast cancer screening worth while in young women?). Population based epidemiological studies are providing the answers to questions of the importance of a given family history (for example, there is about a 70% probability that breast cancer at age 45 in two sisters is due to predisposition, rather than chance). How the genetic information should be used requires careful evaluation in research studies by groups of centres with a special interest. The non-expert clinician faced with such a family should seek the advice of a clinical geneticist.

Genetic changes within tumours

The behaviour of a cancer must presumably be governed by the sum of genetic changes that it contains. It is to be hoped, therefore, that a genetic profile of the tumour will eventually provide a more complete diagnosis and prognosis than conventional pathology. The predictive value of some genetic changes has already been shown —for example in neuroblastoma, where tumours in which the myc oncogene is amplified are more likely to be disseminated and have a poor prognosis, and in breast cancer where amplification of the oncogene erb B2 (her2 or neu) and loss of heterozygosity on chromosome 7 are each associated with worse prognosis.[14] The next challenge will be to move from description to the exploitation of these mutant genes as specific targets for cancer treatment.

1 Nowell PC. Clonal evolution of tumour cell sub-populations. *Science* 1976;**194**:23.
2 *Genetics and cancer*, I and II. In: Cavenee WK, Ponder B, Solomon E, eds. *Cancer surveys*. Vol 9. *Genetic predisposition to cancer*. Oxford: Oxford University Press, 1991.

3 Bishop JM. Molecular themes in oncogenesis. *Cell* 1991;**64**:235-48.
4 Aaronson SA. Growth factors and cancer. *Science* 1991;**254**:1146-53.
5 Weinberg RA. Tumour suppressor genes. *Science* 1991;**254**:1138-46.
6 Knudson AG. Mutation and cancer: statistical study of retinoblastoma. *Proc Natl Acad Sci USA* 1971;**68**:820.
7 Ponder BAJ. Gene losses in human tumours. *Nature* 1988;**335**:400.
8 Easton DF, Peto J. The contribution of inherited predisposition to cancer incidence. In: Cavenee WK, Ponder B, Solomon E, eds. *Cancer surveys*. Vol 9.*Genetic predisposition to cancer*. Oxford: Oxford University Press, 1991:395-416.
9 Ponder BAJ. Genetic predisposition to cancer. *Br J Cancer* 1991;**64**:203-4.
10 Ott J. A short guide to linkage analysis. In: Davies KE, ed. *Human genetic disease: a practical approach*. Oxford: IRL Press, 1986.
11 Nakachi K, Imai K, Hyashi S-I, Watanabe J, Kawajiri K. Genetic susceptibility to squamous cell carcinoma of the lung in relation to cigarette smoking dose. *Cancer Res* 1991;**51**:5177-80.
12 Greene MH, Clarke WH, Tucker MA, Elder DE, Kraemer KH, Guerry D IV, *et al*. Acquired precursors of cutaneous malignant melanoma on the familial dysplastic naevus syndrome. *N Engl J Med* 1985;**312**:91-7.
13 Maher ER, Yates JEW. Familial renal cell carcinoma: clinical and molecular genetic aspects. *Br J Cancer* 1991;**63**:176-9.
14 Bieche I, Champeme MH, Matifas F, Hacene K, Callahan R, Lidereau R. Loss of heterozygosity on chromosome 7q and aggressive primary breast cancer. *Lancet* 1992;**339**: 139-43.

Lung cancer

ROBERT SOUHAMI

In 1985 there were 29 000 cases of lung cancer in men in the United Kingdom and 11 500 in women. The chance of a man getting lung cancer during his life is 8% and for a woman 3%. It is the commonest cancer in men and the third commonest (excluding skin cancer) in women. Even though young people—especially of social classes A, B, and C—are giving up smoking, the habit is still common, and national governments and the European parliament are reluctant to spend money on prevention or to pass effective legislation to reduce cigarette advertising. Nevertheless, there is evidence that the death rate from lung cancer is falling in men aged 20-44,[1] although that in women is not. In the professional lifetime of most of the readers of this article, lung cancer will remain an important cause of death from cancer.

Although the dominant cause of lung cancer is smoking, the disease is curiously diverse histologically and in its clinical behaviour, and management is correspondingly varied. For this reason it is wrong to generalise about treatment and prognosis in lung cancer and, in most cases, there is every reason to seek expert advice.

Biological aspects

The main disease forms and their frequencies are squamous (epidermoid) 50%, adenocarcinoma 15%, large cell (undifferentiated) 10%, and small cell 25%. These frequencies may be changing in the United States and Japan, where adenocarcinoma seems to be predominating in the non-small cell lung cancer category. What is the origin of this curious diversity of histological form? The figure shows a reasonable hypothesis. The cancer inducing event may occur in a

11

pluripotent cell capable of differentiation along different pathways. This might explain why "mixed" tumours (adeno-squamous, small cell-squamous) sometimes occur. Progression of cancer is accompanied by, as in other cancers, genetic change, including mutation in the p53 gene (the product of which is a nuclear phosphoprotein involved in cell division)[2] and a characteristic loss of part of the short arm of chromosome 3 in small cell lung cancer, whose functional significance is unknown.[3] Other genetic changes, which occur more variably, are overexpression of the myc family of oncogenes and abnormalities of the retinoblastoma gene structure or expression. It is not known how these important abnormalities are involved in the origin, or the continuation, of tumour growth.

The different histological types of lung cancer have their counterpart in cell cultures derived from human tumours. Study of these cell culture systems has identified factors which regulate cell growth and has helped to define the particular characteristics of the different tumour types. In cell culture the small cell cancer exhibits a neuroendocrine phenotype. The cells express neural antigens, synthesise and secrete peptide such as antidiuretic and adrenocorticotrophic hormones,[4] and show the sensitivity to cytotoxic drugs that characterises small cell cancer. Several of the peptide hormones (such as gastrin releasing peptide) are secreted by the cell and also bind to the cell surface after secretion. Binding to the surface receptor activates division of the cell that secreted the peptide—so called autocrine growth stimulation.[5] These important growth regulatory mechanisms open up possibilities that we may one day be able to block autocrine stimulation of cell growth as part of a treatment strategy. Adenocarcinoma of the lung may also show some neuroendocrine characteristics in both cell culture and tissue sections, implying again that

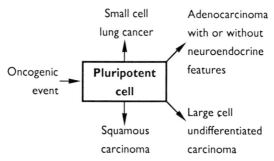

Hypothesis of histological diversity in lung cancer

the distinction between the different morphological types is not absolute.[6]

In tissue culture small cell cancer shows greater chemosensitivity and radiation sensitivity than non-small cell cancer. This distinction is also apparent in the clinic. Nevertheless, the sensitivity of small cell cancer is only relative. Drug and radiation resistance emerge rapidly on treatment. This might be thought to be due to non-small cell elements in the tumour, but in fact there is no good evidence for this. Although treatment of small cell cancer may sometimes result in morphological changes that indicate more epithelial differentiation, there is little evidence that this is related to drug resistance, and the change does not always occur.

The growth in understanding of the biology of lung cancer is welcome as it is already allowing us to think of new therapeutic strategies. These are sorely needed since, although some interesting new developments have occurred in the management of lung cancer, survival for several categories of patients is very poor.

Current management of non-small cell lung cancer

For most patients with non-small cell cancer the best chance of cure comes with an expert resection of a localised tumour. Box 1 gives a simplified staging notation and staging groups. Surgical resection is considered for all stage I and II patients and for some stage III patients. Full staging work up is essential with particular reference to respiratory function, chest wall and mediastinal invasion, and affected adjacent lymph nodes. Full discussion of the criteria for resection is beyond the scope of this article, but assessment of the mediastinum will now include computed tomography and, often, mediastinoscopy or mediastinotomy. For stage I patients (box 1) complete surgical resection is associated with a 50% five year survival, but this figure is higher in those with squamous carcinoma. In stage II cases survival falls to an average of 25% (again slightly higher with squamous cancer).

There is more controversy over the role of surgery in stage III disease, when the tumour may be extending to the chest wall or, more commonly, the hilar nodes are affected. Chances of survival are lessened by larger tumours and affected subcarinal nodes and if mediastinal nodes are affected at more than one level. Even when these adverse features are not present the five year survival is poor (about 25%).

13

Box 1 — TNM staging system and stage grouping for lung cancer

TNM staging system

T 1   Less than 3 cm. Distal to a lobar bronchus
  2   More than 3 cm. More than 2 cm from carina
  3   Any size. Extension into chest wall but not mediastinal
      structures
  4   Affects mediastinum. Pleural effusion

N 0   No regional nodes
  1   Ipsilateral hilum
  2   Ipsilateral mediastinum or subcarina
  3   Contralateral hilum, supraclavicular

M 0/1 Distant metastases absent or present

Stage grouping

I   = T1 or 2, N0
II   = T1 or 2, N1
IIIa = T3, N0 or 1
        T1-3, N2
IIIb = Any T, N3
        T4, any N
IV   = M1, any T, any N

Patients with contralateral mediastinal nodal disease (N3) are not suitable for surgery. Such patients, and those with stage I-IIIa who for other reasons are not fit for surgery, can be considered for radical radiotherapy. The reported results of radiotherapy in these cases have been variable, but a 5 year survival of 6% is a reasonable estimate. Can these results be improved? It is here that an interesting era of clinical research has begun. Three questions remain to be answered conclusively.

Does radiotherapy to the tumour or mediastinum improve the results of surgical resection?

Preoperative radiotherapy has been assessed in several trials. Many of these are old and were too small to be able to show a realistic survival difference. In the largest such collaborative study no benefit was shown,[7] and this was also true in the other smaller studies. Postoperative complications seemed to be more common. Preoperative radiotherapy is often used in the management of the superior sulcus tumour, in which the cancer is at the apex of the lung extending into the neck (Pancoast's syndrome). Moderate doses of radiation are followed by resection three to six weeks later.

Postoperative radiotherapy to the mediastinum has been assessed in a few trials, but all were too small to detect anything but large survival differences. Nevertheless, the trials found no evidence of improved survival, although local recurrence rates were probably reduced.[8] The results of larger studies, such as those being carried out by the Medical Research Council Lung Cancer Working Party, are awaited.

Does chemotherapy improve the results of surgical resection or allow tumours of more advanced stage to be resected?

It is not known if chemotherapy after surgery is beneficial in non-small cell cancer. Response rates to chemotherapy are relatively low (see below) and any survival advantage would probably be small, requiring a large study to show it. A trial by the Lung Cancer Study Group (in the United States) hinted at benefit but was too small to be conclusive. Further trials are needed.

Preoperative chemotherapy is being widely investigated. In uncontrolled trials tumour response rates of 50-70% have been obtained, sometimes allowing resection of a previously unresectable tumour.[9] The resected specimen may show chemotherapy induced necrosis or even no viable tumour. Although these findings are interesting, the contribution to resectability, local control, and survival can be assessed only in randomised trials. Nevertheless, there seem to be grounds for optimism that chemotherapy may help improve the results of surgical resection.

Does chemotherapy improve the results of radical radiotherapy?

Over 20 trials have assessed the value of chemotherapy when added to radiotherapy, and we still do not know the answer despite over 3500 patients having been randomised. Trial design has varied greatly, as has the dose, timing, and nature of the drug treatment. The main reason for our ignorance is, however, that the individual trials have been too small to detect a realistic, small, but important difference. The most recent, and best known, of these trials has been that of the Cancer and Acute Leukaemia Group B.[10] In this study two cycles of cisplatin and vindesine were given before radiotherapy or patients received irradiation alone. Although a significant difference in survival was obtained in favour of the patients treated with chemotherapy, the trial was small and the size of any difference could not be stated with confidence—an important deficiency since a significant difference may be unimportant clinically. In the similar trial of Le Chevalier *et al* systemic metastasis was delayed in the chemotherapy arm and there was a difference in survival in favour of chemotherapy, but the degree was small with overlapping confidence intervals and was not significant.[11] Such small but suggestive studies, however, could miss a 5-10% improvement in survival. Overview analysis of all these trials may help to determine whether survival is improved with chemotherapy, and, most importantly, the size of any benefit.

Over 50% of patients with non-small cell cancer are found to have metastatic disease at presentation. Some of these patients may have symptoms from the primary tumour and others from the metastases, particularly in bone. Radiotherapy is the most effective palliative treatment for local, intrathoracic symptoms such as haemoptysis, bronchial obstruction, and obstruction of the superior vena cava. Recent studies by the Medical Research Council have shown that the radiotherapy fractionation can be simple—17 Gy in two fractions provided as good palliation as 30 Gy in 10 fractions.[12] Bone pain may also be relieved by radiation, and steroids and antibiotics may help anorexia and infections, respectively.

The role of chemotherapy is not well defined. Trials of best supportive care (as outlined above) versus chemotherapy have sometimes shown benefit for chemotherapy in survival,[13] but the differences are small and the clinical value for patients as a whole is debatable. However, some young and fit patients find it difficult to accept a palliative and expectant treatment policy. Furthermore, response rates to chemotherapy are improving and response is often accompanied by improved quality of life.[14] It is not sensible to be dogmatic about this issue. The question is often one of management in its widest sense—physical, social, and psychological—and the experienced oncologist will make different treatment recommendations accordingly.

Current management of small cell lung cancer

Small cell cancer is chemosensitive and radiosensitive and has usually metastasised at presentation. Systemic chemotherapy is therefore the mainstay of treatment. The problem is that the tumour is seldom curable by chemotherapy and relapse is common. In a recent large scale survey the rate of cure was only 3% overall.[15] Adverse prognostic features at presentation include poor performance status, extensive disease, and biochemical abnormalities such as raised alkaline phosphatase or lactic dehydrogenase concentrations or low serum albumin and sodium concentrations.[16] These adverse factors are predictive of early death. If the patient survives and responds to treatment the importance of these factors, present at the time of diagnosis, diminishes with time.

Although the staging notation outlined in box 1 can be applied to small cell cancer, in practice it is usual simply to divide patients into those who have limited disease or extensive disease. Limited means disease confined to one hemithorax, although some definitions allow ipsilateral supraclavicular nodes to be affected. In practice the issue is whether the intrathoracic tumour can be encompassed in a radiation field.

Surgery

An early study suggested that radiation was equivalent to surgery in patients deemed fit for operation by the rather basic criteria of the early 1970s. More refined imaging and staging methods now allow a clearer definition of patients whose tumours may be resectable. Less than 5% of unselected cases would be likely to be candidates for primary surgery.[17] In recent years there has been renewed interest in surgery after initial chemotherapy. In uncontrolled trials patients with limited disease who responded sufficiently to chemotherapy to allow resection (about 15-20% of cases) had an above average survival. However, this is likely to be a form of case selection and only large scale randomised trials will permit evaluation of surgery in this situation. The main problem is systemic disease, and the role of surgery in small cell cancer is likely to remain minor and confined to a small group of selected patients.

Chemotherapy

Small cell cancer responds to a wide variety of chemotherapeutic drugs, and box 2 shows some of the most useful. When drugs are added in combination (box 3) the overall (complete and partial) response rate rises to 70-85%, depending on the stage of disease. The definition of complete response varies. It usually means that there are no symptoms and signs of disease, the chest radiograph appears normal, and if bone or liver scans had given abnormal results these are now normal. If the assessment of response includes a thoracic computed tomogram and bronchoscopy the rate of complete response falls, as would be expected. Complete response occurs in 30-40% of

17

Box 2—Single drugs active in small cell lung cancer

Type of drug	*Examples*
Alkylating agents	Cyclophosphamide, ifosfamide
Platinum analogues	Cisplatin, carboplatin
Epipodophyllotoxins	Etoposide, teniposide
Vinca alkaloids	Vincristine, vindesine
Anthracyclines	Doxorubicin
Antimetabolites	Methotrexate

---

patients with limited stage disease and 20-35% of those with extensive disease. Complete or partial response relieves symptoms caused by cancer. The side effects of chemotherapy are nausea and vomiting, which are better controlled with newer antiemetics; hair loss (with some drugs); and bone marrow suppression with risk of infection. These side effects are a reason for not unduly prolonging chemotherapy. Two large trials[18 19] have shown that there is little advantage in continuing chemotherapy beyond six cycles of treatment, but reduction to four cycles is associated with some diminution in survival.

At present no chemotherapy regimen has been proved superior to others. The combination of etoposide and a platinum drug is widely used, and this may be alternated with cyclophosphamide, doxorubicin, and vincristine (CAV). Evidence conflicts as to the advantage of alternating cycles of chemotherapy, and it probably results in only a minor improvement in median survival.

Intensification of chemotherapy by using weekly treatments, haemopoietic growth factors to support the white cell count, or high dose chemotherapy with autologous bone marrow support have not yet been shown to improve survival. As in other aspects of treatment

---

Box 3—Commonly used drug combinations in small cell lung cancer

Cyclophosphamide, doxorubicin, vincristine
Cisplatin, etoposide
Cyclophosphamide, doxorubicin, etoposide
Cyclophosphamide, methotrexate, lomustine, vincristine

---

of lung cancer improvements in survival are likely to be small and large scale trials are necessary.

Radiotherapy

The role of thoracic radiotherapy in limited disease has been assessed by several clinical trials. These have tended to show a benefit from its use,[20] and a recent overview analysis has confirmed an improvement of about 5% in two year survival. The optimum dose, schedule, and timing are uncertain. Doses of 50-55 Gy are commonly used, given in 20-25 daily fractions. Recently there has been interest in combining chemotherapy and radiotherapy so that the two modalities are given concurrently early in treatment. The toxicity is more severe, but high local control rates have been reported.

Prophylactic irradiation of the brain has been widely advocated to prevent the development of clinically apparent brain metastasis. This is achieved, but at the cost of some short term and long term toxicity. Survival does not seem to be prolonged as this is determined by control of disease at other sites, and the relative merits and disadvantages of brain irradiation remain debatable.

Future developments in management of small cell lung cancer

Future directions in small cell cancer will be the exploration of new methods of increasing the intensity of chemotherapy and further exploration of radiotherapy and chemotherapy combinations. The development of drugs that interfere with autocrine growth stimulation seems certain, along with new cytotoxic drugs. Radioactive monoclonal antibodies directed to the neural antigens on the cell surface may be a means of administering systemic radiotherapy after remission has been achieved with chemotherapy. In each case the lengthy process of early small scale studies followed by large scale trials will be necessary. There are many questions still to be answered and we can be reasonably optimistic that, slowly, a significant improvement in survival will be achieved.

1 Doll R. Are we winning the fight against cancer? An epidemiological assessment. *Eur J Cancer* 1990;**26**:500-8.
2 Iggo R, Gatter K, Bartek J, Lane D, Harris AL. Increased expression of mutant forms of p53 oncogene in primary lung cancer. *Lancet* 1990;**335**: 675-9.

3 Whang-Peng J, Bunn PA, Kao-Shan CS, Lee EC, Carney DN, Gazdar AF, *et al.* Specific chromosome defect associated with human small cell lung cancer: deletion 3p (14-23). *Science* 1982;**215**:181-2.

4 Carney DN, De Leij L. Lung cancer biology. *Seminars in Oncology* 1988;**15**: 199-214.

5 Cuttitta F, Carney DN, Mulshine J, Moody TW, Fedorko J, Fischler A, *et al.* Bombesin-like peptides can function as autocrine growth factors in human small cell lung cancer. *Nature* 1985;**316**:823-6.

6 Linnoila RI, Mulshine JL, Steinberg SM, Funa K, Matthews MJ, Cotelingham JD, *et al.* Neuroendocrine differentiation in endocrine and nonendrocrine lung carcinomas. *Am J Clin Pathol* 1988;**90**:641-52.

7 National Cancer Institutes Collaborative Intergroup Study: Preoperative irradiation of cancer of the lung. Final report of a therapeutic trial. *Cancer* 1975;**36**:914-25.

8 Lung Cancer Study Group. Effects of post-operative mediastinal radiation on completely resected stage II and stage III epidermoid cancer of the lung. *N Engl J Med* 1986;**315**:1377-81.

9 Kris MG, Gralla RJ, Martini N, Stampleman LV, Burke MJ. Pre-operative and adjuvant chemotherapy in locally advanced non-small cell lung cancer. *Surg Clin North Am* 1987;**67**:1051-8.

10 Dillman RO, Seagren SL, Propert KJ, Guerra J, Eaton WL, Perry MC, *et al.* A randomized trial of induction chemotherapy plus high dose radiation versus radiation alone in stage III non-small-cell lung cancer. *N Engl J Med* 1990;**323**:940-5.

11 Le Chevalier T, Arriagada R, Quoix E, Ruffie P, Martin M, Tarage M, *et al.* Radiotherapy alone versus combined chemotherapy and radiotherapy in non-resectable non-small cell lung cancer. First analysis of a randomized trial in 353 patients. *J Natl Cancer Inst* 1991;**83**:417-23.

12 Medical Research Council Lung Cancer Working Party. Inoperable non-small cell lung cancer (NSCLC): a Medical Research Council randomised trial of palliative radiotherapy with two fractions or ten fractions. *Br J Cancer* 1991;**63**:265-70.

13 Rapp E, Pater JL, Willan A, Cormier Y, Murray N, Evans WK, *et al.* Chemotherapy can prolong survival in patients with advanced non-small-cell lung cancer—report of a Canadian multicenter randomized trial. *J Clin Oncol* 1988;**6**:633-41.

14 Cullen MH, Joshi R, Chetiyawardana AD, Woodroffe CM. Mitomycin, ifosfamide and cis-platin in non-small lung cancer: treatment good enough to compare. *Br J Cancer* 1988;**58**: 359-61.

15 Souhami RL, Law K. Longevity in small cell lung cancer. *Br J Cancer* 1990;**61**:584-9.

16 Souhami RL, Bradbury I, Geddes DM, Spiro SG, Harper PG, Tobias JS. The prognostic significance of laboratory parameters measured at diagnosis in small cell carcinoma of the lung. *Cancer Res* 1985;**45**:2878-82.

17 Østerlind K, Hansen M, Hansen HH, Dombernowsky P. Influence of surgical resection prior to chemotherapy on the long-term results in small cell lung cancer: a study of 150 operable patients. *Eur J Cancer Clin Oncol* 1986;**22**:589-93.

18 Spiro SG, Souhami RL, Geddes DM, Ash CM, Quinn H, Harper PG, *et al.* Duration of chemotherapy in small cell lung cancer: a Cancer Research Campaign trial. *Br J Cancer* 1989;**59**:578-83.

19 Medical Research Council Lung Cancer Working Party. Controlled trial of twelve versus six courses of chemotherapy in the treatment of small cell lung cancer. *Br J Cancer* 1989;**59**: 584-90.

20 Perry MC, Walter LE, Propert KJ, Ware JH, Zimmer B, Chahinian AP, *et al.* Chemotherapy with or without radiation therapy in limited small-cell carcinoma of the lung. *New Engl J Med* 1987;**316**:912-8.

Early breast cancer

R D RUBENS

Breast cancer is Britain's most common malignancy in women, estimated to affect one in 12 of the female population. About 80% of women present with apparently localised disease which is surgically resectable: so called early breast cancer. Nevertheless, in about half relapse occurs despite intended curative treatment. Controversy about the treatment of early breast cancer has existed for at least a century and continues. Two questions have predominated. Firstly, is mastectomy necessary or can the affected breast safely be preserved? Secondly, can adjuvant systemic therapy eliminate micrometastatic disease present, but not identifiable, at diagnosis, and if so how should patients best be selected for such treatment? The available evidence on these issues is considered and a reasonable approach to present good practice is described.

Definition of early breast cancer

The term early breast cancer describes disease which, at presentation and after initial assessment, is apparently confined to the breast and deemed to be technically resectable; axillary lymph nodes may be palpable. The cancer is operable if clinical examination excludes extension of the primary tumour or axillary node metastases to either the skin or the chest wall and confirms that there is no supraclavicular lymphadenopathy. In other words, signs of locally advanced disease are absent. Ancillary investigations, aiming at identifying potential distant metastases, normally include haematological and biochemical tests and chest radiography. If these produce normal results many doctors consider further investigation unnecessary. However, isotopic bone scanning to screen for skeletal metastases is often routinely performed, but the low positive predictive value has called into question the cost effectiveness of this investigation.[1]

The term early to describe operable breast cancer is often a misnomer as the low resolution of staging tests means that occult metastatic disease is not identified in many patients. The risk of distant metastatic disease is particularly high when axillary lymph nodes are affected. It is useful to designate the disease as stage I when the axillary nodes are not affected and stage II when they are. Assigning this staging on clinical grounds is extremely unreliable and it is best done after the true axillary node status has been determined histopathologically.[2] Once determined, this staging and its correlation with occult metastatic disease assist in the rational selection of systemic treatment as part of the composite management of early breast cancer. The figure shows the comparative prognostic implications for the two stages and how they contrast with those for stages III (locally advanced disease) and IV (distant metastases).

After early breast cancer has been defined the principles for treatment are clear: *eradication of locoregional disease* in a way that enables *estimation of risk of relapse* for the effective *selection of adjuvant systemic treatment.*

Locoregional treatment

The above aims are achieved effectively by modified radical mastectomy, whereby the breast is removed in continuity with the axillary contents. Unlike in the classic Halsted operation, the pectoralis major is left intact, although the pectoralis minor is sometimes removed to

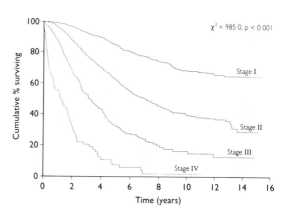

Survival of patients with breast cancer from diagnosis according to stage of disease at presentation (from the database of Imperial Cancer Research Fund clinical oncology unit, Guy's Hospital)

$\chi^2 = 985 \cdot 0, p < 0.001$

permit complete dissection of the axilla. The procedure gives a high probability of control of local disease, and recurrence in the axilla is rare. Postoperative radiotherapy is unnecessary and only increases the risk of lymphoedema of the arm. Full information on axillary node status is obtained, and complete removal of the tumour provides adequate tissue for histopathological examination and other tests such as flow cytometry and steroid receptor analysis to help plan further treatment. The main drawback of this approach is loss of the breast, although this can partly be compensated for by reconstructive procedures.

Alternatives to mastectomy

Is it possible to fulfil all the objectives of primary treatment without the need for mastectomy? The first test of breast conserving treatment in a prospective clinical trial showed it to be less satisfactory than radical mastectomy.[3] The method entailed wide excision of the primary tumour followed by radiotherapy to the breast and the draining lymph node areas. Local recurrence was high and associated with a higher incidence of distant metastases. By modern standards the postoperative dose of radiation to the axilla was too low, and the trial highlighted the importance of achieving local control of the disease. The technique also omitted axillary dissection and so failed to provide the prognostic information now considered important for planning adjuvant treatment (see below). Greater success was achieved in the Milan trial, in which quadrantectomy, not dissimilar to wide excision, combined with axillary clearance and radiotherapy to the preserved breast was compared with radical mastectomy.[4] Locoregional control was satisfactory and the subsequent incidence of distant metastases and survival were identical in the two arms of the trial. Thus breast conservation was shown to be safe, provided that locoregional control was adequate, and could be combined with axillary clearance to give an additional therapeutic advantage and provide important prognostic information.

The principal disadvantage of the above techniques of breast conserving surgery is that wide excision, particularly with large tumours and small breasts, often gives unsatisfactory cosmetic results. Further work was therefore done to permit removal of only the macroscopic tumour without a margin of apparently normal breast tissue. To achieve this objective without compromising safety it was recognised that radiation doses to the conserved breast would need to be high and that this, in itself, could prevent a good cosmetic outcome because of skin reactions and fibrosis. To overcome this difficulty external beam radiotherapy to the whole breast has been combined with interstitial implantation of radioactive sources (brachytherapy) to the tumour bed to achieve higher irradiation of the site of the tumour but not to the skin.[5] The technique was developed further at Guy's Hospital, where after histological diagnosis by needle biopsy a single operative procedure comprised axillary clearance, excision of the tumour, and implantation of tubes into the tumour bed for subsequent loading with radioactive iridium.[6] The iridium boost was given immediately postoperatively and was followed by external beam treatment to the breast. This technique, which gives excellent cosmetic results in most patients, has now been compared with modified radical mastectomy in a prospective randomised clinical trial. Locoregional recurrence, distant relapse, and survival were the same for the two treatments.[7] Thus it seems clear that, with adequate radiotherapy, breast conservation is a safe alternative to mastectomy.

Problems with conservation

Although breast conservation fulfils all the objectives of primary treatment, relapse in the conserved breast is a potential problem. Unfortunately, this risk is higher in younger women, those for whom breast conservation is probably most important. Nevertheless, many women remain free from breast recurrence after conservation surgery, and even in the event of recurrence mastectomy is usually feasible and long term prognosis does not seem to be compromised.[8] Although preservation of body image is clearly better after breast conservation than after mastectomy, psychological morbidity is similar after both procedures, indicating that patients are most concerned about the presence of cancer rather than loss of the breast.[9]

A further disadvantage of current conservation techniques is the long duration of postoperative radiotherapy. Techniques are therefore being developed to enable most, and possibly all, of the radiotherapy to be given by brachytherapy. A pilot study has shown that it is practicable to give high doses of radiotherapy by iridium implantation alone over a few days.[10] Should this technique be validated and developed by using other isotopes such as caesium to reduce treatment times further, breast conservation could become widely applicable to most patients irrespective of age. Short radiation treatment times would also overcome the problem of how best to combine and schedule radiotherapy with adjuvant chemotherapy.

Conservation techniques are unsatisfactory for large operable tumours and tend to be restricted to tumours less than 4 cm in diameter. In a high proportion of patients with larger tumours who desire breast conservation, tumour size can be reduced by primary chemotherapy to enable breast conserving surgery.[11]

The conservation techniques discussed so far have incorporated complete removal of the primary tumour and axillary clearance. But there has been much experience, particularly in France, of treating breast cancer conservatively by radiotherapy with minimal surgical interference other than biopsy. Long follow up of these studies is available and there is no evidence to suggest that long term outcome has been unfavourable.[12 13] However, little comparative information from clinical trials is available, and with the current demand for histopathological information, particularly on axillary node status, for planning treatment these approaches are not entirely satisfactory.

Risk evaluation

The most powerful predictor of outcome after primary surgery is the degree to which axillary lymph nodes are affected. Prognosis steadily worsens as the number of axillary lymph nodes affected increases.[14] The risk of relapse needs to be estimated to enable rational decisions on the selection of adjuvant systemic treatment. Originally, adjuvant treatment was reserved for patients with affected axillary nodes, but both stage I and stage II disease can now be subdivided into different prognostic subsets by considering other factors such as the size of the primary tumour, histopathological features, and indices of proliferative activity of tumour cells. Flow cytometry permits estimation of ploidy and S phase fraction; multivariate analysis shows the S phase fraction to be a covariate independent of tumour size and axillary node status but not of histopathological grade.[15] Although flow cytometry requires specialised equipment and technical expertise, it gives a more objective index of prognosis than histopathological grading, which is particularly observer dependent.

Application of tumour size and measurements of S phase fraction to patients with node negative disease allows the definition of three distinct subgroups: firstly, those with a good prognosis, having survival expectancy similar to that of the unaffected age matched female population; secondly, an intermediate risk group with a 20% chance of recurrence at five years; and, thirdly, a poor prognosis group having an outlook similar to those with one to three positive nodes—namely, a 50% chance of recurrence at five years.[16] In node

25

positive disease, those with four or more nodes affected have a significantly worse prognosis than those with one to three nodes affected, but consideration of histological type and grade can refine prediction further (table I). Several other markers of prognosis have been described, but none has so far found a routine practical role. Steroid receptor concentrations, which have clear predictive value for endocrine therapy of advanced disease, are not powerful predictors of prognosis in the early disease.[17]

Other factors which may influence the clinical course of breast cancer include the timing of surgery in relation to menstruation in premenopausal patients[18] and the occurrence of severe psychosocial stress.[19] These observations point the way to investigating the probable underlying endocrinological and immunological mechanisms, which should in due course help to identify new therapeutic interventions.

Adjuvant systemic treatment

The aim of adjuvant systemic treatment is to eradicate micrometastatic disease. The eradication cannot be observed directly, and evidence for the efficacy of adjuvant endocrine treatment or chemotherapy relies on data from clinical trials. These studies provided early evidence that adjuvant treatment significantly delayed relapse, a finding not unexpected with treatments effective at inducing regres-

TABLE I—Prognostic subsets in operable breast cancer

Subset	No of axillary nodes affected	Other discriminants	Chance of being relapse free at 5 years
1	None	Diameter <1 cm	95%
2	None	Diameter ≥1 cm Favourable histology or S phase fraction <10%	80%
3	None	Diameter ≥1 cm Unfavourable histology or S phase fraction ≥10%	50%
4	1-3	Any histology	50%
5	≥4	Favourable histology	50%
6	≥4	Unfavourable histology	<25%

Favourable histology=ductal grade I, tubular, mucoid.
Unfavourable histology=ductal grades II and III, lobular, medullary.

sion of advanced disease. There was, however, considerable debate over whether adjuvant systemic treatment influenced survival, because clinical trials produced apparently inconsistent results. Eventually it became clear that the controversy was consequent on heterogeneity among trials in entry criteria, type of adjuvant treatment, follow up procedures, and treatments used on relapse. Moreover, most trials were not large enough to identify small but significant differences.

The problem was overcome by using meta-analysis, which has essentially ended the conflict over whether or not adjuvant systemic treatment affects survival.[20] It has now been shown beyond reasonable doubt that in most prognostic subsets of patients with breast cancer either endocrine therapy or chemotherapy reduces the annual odds of death by about 25%, thus avoiding about 10% of deaths at 10 years after diagnosis. The most recent meta-analysis is based on information from 133 randomised trials involving 75 000 women.[20] Such large numbers not only give firm evidence of the general efficacy of adjuvant treatment but also enable separate analyses on different groups of patients and for different types of treatment.

In patients less than 50 years old chemotherapy has become established as having the clearest effect in reducing the annual odds of death. Prolonged multiple drug treatment—for example, with cyclophosphamide, methotrexate, and 5-fluorouracil (CMF)—is more effective than either limited perioperative chemotherapy or prolonged single agent treatment; treatment beyond four to six months does not enhance the effect. Similarly, the current meta-analysis also shows that ovarian ablation confers a similar reduction in death rate.

In older, predominantly postmenopausal women, tamoxifen leads to a highly significant reduction in the annual odds of death; the size of the effect increases with rising concentrations of oestrogen receptor in the primary tumour. The optimal duration of tamoxifen treatment is not yet known, but present results favour prolonged use—at least two years. The effect of chemotherapy in postmenopausal women has been controversial. The meta-analysis shows a positive therapeutic effect, but it is considerably less than for tamoxifen, which, given its considerably fewer side effects compared with chemotherapy, remains the standard adjuvant systemic treatment for postmenopausal patients.

Cost effectiveness of adjuvant treatment

It is now certain that adjuvant treatment by either endocrine

27

or chemotherapeutic means produces a significant, but relatively modest, reduction in the death rate from breast cancer. If these treatments are to be used most effectively it is necessary realistically to estimate the expectations from them in different prognostic subsets of patients. Consider, for example, a hypothetical subgroup of patients with an 80% five year survival expectancy. A treatment which reduces the five year mortality by 25% would lead to just 5% of deaths being avoided at this time point at the expense of 95% of patients being treated without benefit (table II). On the other hand, if the five year survival expectancy was only 20% then in 100 patients 20 deaths would be avoided but 80 patients would still have been treated without benefit. For a non-toxic treatment such as tamoxifen there is little disadvantage other than the economic cost of patients being overtreated, but for a toxic treatment, like chemotherapy, the cost-benefit considerations become more finely balanced. Even if we had a more effective adjuvant treatment which reduced the five year mortality by 50%, we would still find that as many as 60% of patients would be treated without benefit in the worst prognostic category in table II.

In judging the effective use of adjuvant treatment it is necessary to consider not only its efficacy but also the potential adverse long term consequences. Tamoxifen, being an antioestrogen, could theoretically have deleterious effects on lipid and bone metabolism, predisposing to coronary artery disease and osteoporosis. Fortunately, data suggest that for both bone and lipid metabolism, tamoxifen has an oestrogen agonist effect.[21][22] There is concern that this could increase the risk of endometrial cancer, but this is unlikely to outweigh the

TABLE II—Effect of hypothetical treatment that reduces five year mortality by 25% (or 50%) in 100 patients

No of patients	Expected 5 year survival without treatment			
	80%	60%	40%	20%
Expected to be alive without treatment (a)	80	60	40	20
Expected dead without treatment	20	40	60	80
Dead at 5 years with treatment (b)	15 (10)	30 (20)	45 (30)	60 (40)
Avoiding deaths	5 (10)	10 (20)	15 (30)	20 (40)
Treated without benefit ($a+b$)	95 (90)	90 (80)	85 (70)	80 (60)

28

TABLE III—Guide to adjuvant systemic treatment for early breast cancer

Tumour characteristic	Prognostic subset (table I)	Adjuvant treatment	
		Premenopausal patients	Postmenopausal patients
Node negative, low risk	1	None	None
Node negative, intermediate risk	2	Ovarian ablation or tamoxifen	Tamoxifen
Node negative, high risk	3	Chemotherapy	Tamoxifen
Node positive, low risk	4,5	Chemotherapy	Tamoxifen
Node positive, high risk	6	Trials of intensive chemotherapy in research centres	Tamoxifen

substantial benefits of adjuvant tamoxifen.[23] Adjuvant chemotherapy has, so far, been free from long term adverse effects,[24] although the increasing use of anthracyclines must be viewed cautiously for potential cardiomyopathic effects.

Balancing the benefits of adjuvant treatment against adverse effects can be difficult, particularly when it is recognised that many patients will be treated without benefit. A method has been described to calculate the time patients spend without symptoms from either recurrent disease or the toxic effects of therapy, which helps to make comparisons with patients not given adjuvant treatment.[25] The method has been refined further to enable quality to be adjusted for by applying utility coefficients to each time component. Experience with this technique is still limited, but it provides a potentially useful approach to cost-benefit analysis for adjuvant treatment. For the present, table III gives a reasonable framework within which to use adjuvant treatment.

Conclusion

Much evidence supports the view that breast cancer can be treated both radically and safely in many, but not all, patients by breast conserving techniques. Adjuvant systemic therapy has been shown convincingly to reduce mortality from this disease significantly. Nevertheless, there is a continuing need for more effective treatments to be developed together with improved methods of selecting patients for them on the basis of precise prognostic indices. These aims would be greatly facilitated if women with breast cancer were, as far as possible, treated in prospective controlled clinical trials.

EARLY BREAST CANCER

1 Coleman RE, Rubens RD, Fogelman I. Reappraisal of the baseline bone scan in breast cancer. *J Nucl Med* 1988;**29**:1045-9.
2 Davies GC, Millis RR, Hayward JL. Assessment of axillary lymph node status. *Ann Surg* 1980;**192**:148-51.
3 Atkins HJ, Hayward JL, Klugman DJ, Wayte AB. Treatment of early breast cancer: a report after ten years of a clinical trial. *BMJ* 1972;ii:423-9.
4 Veronesi U, Banti A, Del Vecchio, Saccozzi R, Clemente C, Greco M, *et al*. Comparison of Halsted mastectomy with quadrantectomy, axillary dissection and radiotherapy in early breast cancer: long-term results. *Eur J Cancer Clin Oncol* 1986;**22**:1085-9.
5 Pierquin B, Owen R, Maylin C, Otmezguine Y, Raynal M, Mueller W, *et al*. Radical radiation therapy of breast cancer. *Int J Radiat Oncol Biol Phys* 1980;**6**:17-24.
6 Hayward JL, Winter PJ, Tong D, Rubens RD, Payne JG, Chaudary MA, *et al*. A new combined approach to the conservative treatment of early breast cancer. *Surgery* 1984;**95**:270-4.
7 Fentiman IS. *Detection and treatment of early breast cancer*. London: Martin Dunitz, 1990:79-82.
8 Fisher B, Anderson S, Fisher ER, Redmond C, Wickerham DL, Wolmark N, *et al*. Significance of ipsilateral breast tumour recurrence after lumpectomy. *Lancet* 1991;**338**:327-31.
9 Fallowfield LJ, Baum M, Maguire GP. Effects of breast conservation on psychological morbidity associated with the diagnosis and treatment of early breast cancer. *BMJ* 1986;**293**:1331-4.
10 Fentiman IS, Poole C, Tong D, Winter PJ, Mayles HMO, Turner P, *et al*. Iridium implant treatment without external radiotherapy for operable breast cancer: a pilot study. *Eur J Cancer* 1991;**27**:447-50.
11 Bonadonna G, Veronesi U, Brambilla C, Ferrari L, Luini A, Greco M, *et al*. Primary chemotherapy to avoid mastectomy in tumours with diameters of three centimeters or more. *J Natl Cancer Inst* 1990;**82**:1539-45.
12 Calle R, Pilleron JP, Schlienger P, Vilcoq JR. Conservative management of operable breast cancer. Ten years experience at the Foundation Curie. *Cancer* 1978;**42**:2045-53.
13 Amalric R, Santamaria F, Robert F, Seigle J, Altschuler C, Kurtz JM, *et al*. Radiation therapy with or without primary limited surgery for operable breast cancer. A 20 year experience at the Marseilles Cancer Institute. *Cancer* 1982;**49**:30-4.
14 Nemoto T, Vana J, Bedwani RN, Management and survival of female breast cancer: results of a national survey by the American College of Surgeons. *Cancer* 1980;**45**:2917-24.
15 O'Reilly SM, Camplejohn RS, Barnes DM, Millis RR, Allen D, Rubens RD, *et al*. DNA index, S-phase fraction, histological grade and prognosis in breast cancer. *Br J Cancer* 1990;**61**:671-4.
16 O'Reilly SM, Camplejohn RS, Barnes DM, Millis RR, Rubens RD, Richards MA. Node negative breast cancer: prognostic subgroups defined by tumour size and flow cytometry. *J Clin Oncol* 1990;**8**:2040-6.
17 Stewart JF, Rubens RD, Millis RM, King RJ, Hayward JL. Steroid receptors and prognosis in operable (stage I and II) breast cancer. *Eur J Cancer Clin Oncol* 1983;**19**:1381-7.
18 Badwe RA, Gregory WM, Chaudary MA, Richards MA, Bentley AE, Rubens RD, *et al*. Timing of surgery during menstrual cycle and survival of premenopausal women with operable breast cancer. *Lancet* 1991;**337**:1261-4.
19 Ramirez AJ, Craig TKJ, Watson JP, Fentimen IS, North WRS, Rubens RD. Stress and relapse of breast cancer. *BMJ* 1989;**298**:291-3.
20 Early Breast Cancer Trialists' Collaborative Group. Systemic treatment of early breast cancer by hormonal, cytotoxic, or immune therapy. *Lancet* 1992;**339**:71-85.
21 Love RR, Mazess RB, Tormey DC, Barden HS, Newcomb PA, Jordan VC. Bone mineral density in women with breast cancer treated for at least two years with tamoxifen. *Breast Cancer Res Treat* 1988;**12**:297-302.
22 McDonald CC, Stewart HJ (for the Scottish Breast Cancer Committee). Fatal myocardial infarction in the Scottish adjuvant tamoxifen trial. *BMJ* 1991;**303**:435-7.
23 Andersson M, Storm HH, Mouridsen HT. Incidence of new primary cancers after adjuvant tamoxifen therapy and radiotherapy for early breast cancer. *J Natl Cancer Inst* 1991;**83**:1013-7.
24 Holdener EE, Nissen-Meyer R, Bonadonna G, Jones SE, Howell A, Rubens RD, *et al*. Second malignant neoplasms in operable carcinoma of the breast. In: Senn HJ, ed. *Recent results in cancer research: adjuvant chemotherapy of breast cancer (No 96)* Berlin, Heidelberg: Springer-Verlag 1984:188-96.
25 Goldhirsch A, Gelber RD, Castiglione M (for the International Breast Cancer Study Group). Adjuvant therapy of breast cancer. *Eur J Cancer* 1991;**27**: 389-99.

Testicular cancer and related neoplasms

G M MEAD

This chapter is primarily concerned with germ cell tumours of the testis (seminoma and teratoma), which are by far the most common testicular cancers in adults. Comparable neoplasms may, however, develop in the ovary or at extragonadal sites, particularly the mediastinum in men and the pineal area in both sexes. Primary retroperitoneal tumours are probably rare; testicular biopsy specimens from patients with these tumours often show histological changes that suggest that the testis was in fact the primary site.

Germ cell tumours of the testis are comparatively rare, comprising about 1% of cancers in men; however, they are by far the commonest cause of cancer in young men (table I) and their incidence has

TABLE I—Incidence of four most common cancers in men aged 15-34

Site	No of cancers/ year*
Testis	485
Hodgkin's disease	255
Malignant brain tumours	155
Leukaemia	146

*Office of Population Censuses and Surveys cancer statistics registrations, England and Wales, 1985.

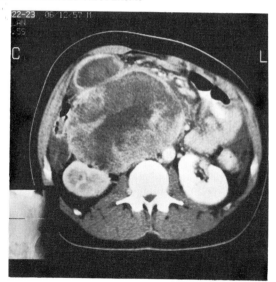

Figure 1—Computed tomogram of large cystic retroperitoneal mass which was the presenting feature in 33 year old man. No testicular primary tumour was palpable. Concentrations of tumour markers were greatly raised (α fetoprotein 30 300 U/l; chorionic gonadotrophin 780 U/l (normal <10)). Ultrasonography showed a tumour in the right testis

increased rapidly in the Western world,[1] as has the incidence of ovarian germ cell malignancy.

During the past 15 years management of these tumours has become highly sophisticated, and patients in whom prognosis was hopeless only 15 years ago are now commonly cured. These advances are largely due to chemotherapy, particularly with cisplatin and its derivatives.[2] The production of the tumour markers α fetoprotein and human chorionic gonadotrophin by these cancers is of particular importance, and they have served as a model in the search for similar markers in other tumour types.

Though most men with a germ cell tumour present with an obvious testicular mass, this is not always the case. Indeed a diagnosis of metastatic germ cell tumour needs to be excluded in any young man presenting with metastatic cancer in whom no obvious primary site is present (fig 1). This diagnosis can usually be effectively excluded by measurement of tumour markers, together with testicular ultrasonography and a review of the diagnostic biopsy specimen. No patient with a putative germ cell tumour, however ill at presentation, should be considered beyond cure. Most such patients are now managed by specialist units.

TABLE II—Incidence of testicular cancer in England and Wales

Year	No of cases*	Rate/ 100 000 population
1970	660	2·7
1975	762	3·2
1980	843	3·5
1985	922	3·8

*Office of Population Censuses and Surveys cancer statistics registrations.

Epidemiology

In England and Wales 900-1000 new cases of testicular germ cell tumours are seen each year (representing a lifetime risk of about 1 in 500). There has been a remarkable 300% increase in incidence in men aged 25-29 during this century, and the numbers continue to rise (table II). The main risk factors are a history of unilateral or bilateral testicular maldescent (recorded in about 10% of cases of testicular cancer) or a strong family history. It is not known why testicular cancer is increasing in incidence. At present public health measures include encouraging early identification of cancers by public education and correction of maldescent (although the impact of this on the future incidence of cancer is unknown).

Pathogenesis

Testicular germ cell tumours are often histologically intimately related to areas of in situ germ cell carcinoma, and these lesions are thought to precede germ cell cancer in a high proportion of cases.[3] Testicular biopsy has shown carcinoma in situ in a proportion of patients with cryptorchidism or gonadal dysgenesis and in the contralateral testis of patients with a germ cell tumour. The risk of subsequent germ cell tumour in patients with carcinoma in situ may be as high as 50%.[4] These histological lesions can, however, be eradicated with radiotherapy.

Malignant teratoma

Malignant teratomas (or non-seminomatous germ cell tumours) comprise about 50% of testicular germ cell cancers. They occur in younger men, median age 25-30. These tumours are histologically diverse and often include various malignant and benign (teratoma differentiated) elements. In particular, recognisable areas of seminoma, trophoblastic tissue (the source of chorionic gonadotrophin), yolk sac tumour (the source of α fetoprotein), and undifferentiated elements may be present. The differentiated elements comprise mature tissues and commonly include glandular structures and cartilage. All these neoplastic elements may be present in pure form, and all are capable of metastasis.

Clinical management

About 90% of patients with malignant teratoma have an obvious primary tumour in the testis. In the remaining cases the primary tumour may be occult (and can often be visualised by testicular ultrasonography), missed, or absent (extragonadal primary). About 80% of patients presenting with testicular teratoma have raised concentrations of α fetoprotein or chorionic gonadotrophin, or both. Such patients should have sequential measurements of serum markers after orchidectomy together with computed tomography of the chest and abdomen. If the scan gives normal results and the concentrations of the markers fall to or remain normal the patient is regarded as having stage I disease.

Stage I teratoma

Stage I teratoma comprises around 50% of cases. Traditionally these patients have been managed with radiotherapy (in Britain) or retroperitoneal lymph node dissection (in the United States). However, in recent years the accepted approach in Britain has been a "watch" policy with careful sequential review. Only 25-30% of patients managed in this fashion develop metastatic disease, usually within a year (though late relapses are well described), and almost all will be cured with combinations of chemotherapeutic drugs including cisplatin.[5] Recent studies have focused on identifying patients at high risk of relapse by careful review of the histology of the primary tumour.[6] Venous invasion in the primary tumour together with several other histological features have clearly been shown to be important risk factors, and trials are in progress to see if patients in

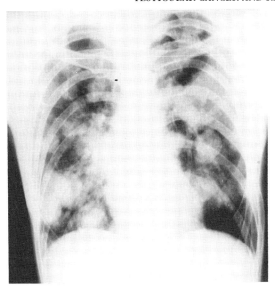

Figure 2—Severe lung metastases in 33 year old man presenting with testicular mass, gynaecomastia, and haemoptysis. Chorionic gonadotrophin concentration was 26 600 U/l (normal <10)

these groups can be spared the risk of relapse by receiving initial limited chemotherapy.

Metastatic disease

Malignant teratoma metastasises in an unpredictable fashion. Para-aortic nodal metastases often occur first, but nodal disease in the chest and neck and lung metastases are also common at presentation. Histologically, these metastases are diverse and may contain any of the possible elements in the primary tumour.

Occasionally the presentation is fulminant, particularly when elements of choriocarcinoma predominate, when extensive lung (fig 2) and other visceral metastases are often present, commonly in conjunction with haemoptysis and gynaecomastia.[7]

In Britain all patients with metastatic disease are treated with combination chemotherapy (in the United States low volume para-aortic disease is still treated surgically). Cure rates are high—in a recent Medical Research Council retrospective study 85% of patients were alive three years after treatment.[8] Management of these patients is complex, often comprising a mixture of chemotherapy for the frankly malignant components of the disease and surgery—often multisite—for any residual masses. These commonly contain differentiated elements (which if left untreated may grow, become un-

35

differentiated, or become malignant) but may also be entirely necrotic or contain active cancer.[9]

The type and intensity of chemotherapy needed is determined from known prognostic factors. In particular, bulky disease (for example, abdominal masses >10 cm, more than 20 lung metastases), disease present in the liver or central nervous system, or the presence of high marker concentrations (α fetoprotein >1000 U/l, chorionic gonadotrophin >10 000 U/l) may indicate a need for more intensive and prolonged chemotherapy.[8]

The standard chemotherapy for the two thirds of cases without adverse features is bleomycin, etoposide, and cisplatin (BEP), given for four courses at three weekly intervals and followed by surgery if necessary.[10] At least 90% of such patients are curable. This treatment is relatively toxic and recent trials have explored lower toxicity treatments with the aim of improving tolerance of treatment without loss of efficacy. These trials have included the use of three versus four courses of treatment,[11] substitution of carboplatin for cisplatin,[12] and attempts to reduce or omit the bleomycin component of the drug combination.

About 60-70% of patients with a poor prognosis are at present curable. Trials in these patients are directed at improving results of treatment, usually by using more intensive and thereby more toxic chemotherapy.[13 14] A recent study in such patients compared standard bleomycin, etoposide, and cisplastin with a new form of this regimen containing a high dose of cisplatin.[13] Despite increased toxicity no improvement in survival was seen. A study in Britain and Europe is currently comparing bleomycin, etoposide, and cisplatin with a more intensive treatment, BOP/VIP (bleomycin, vincristine, and cisplatin followed by etoposide, ifosfamide, and cisplatin).[14] This study incorporates the haemopoietic growth factor granulocyte colony stimulating factor as part of the randomisation. It is hoped that this drug will enable more chemotherapy to be given.

Most patients with poor prognosis teratoma will require a laparotomy or thoracotomy at completion of treatment to remove residual mass lesions (fig 3).

Seminoma of the testis

Testicular seminoma comprises about 50% of cases. These cancers occur at a median age of 35-40 but may present at any point in adult life. Seminoma can produce chorionic gonadotrophin in relatively

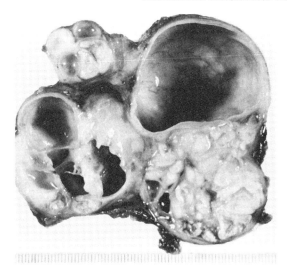

Figure 3—Large mass of differentiated teratoma resected from the retroperitoneum of 19 year old man after chemotherapy

small quantities, together with placental alkaline phosphatase. Metastatic potential is low for many of these tumours, and at presentation about 75% of men have no evidence of metastatic disease (stage I). Traditionally such patients have been treated with prophylactic radiotherapy to the ipsilateral para-aortic and pelvic lymph nodes—a well tolerated and highly successful approach for these radiosensitive tumours—with relapse rates under 5% and cure almost the rule.[15] The need for radiotherapy has recently been questioned, and a few centres have adopted a watch policy, reserving treatment for relapse of disease.[16] About 15% of patients in these studies have relapsed and have required chemo-therapy. Relapse often occurs relatively late and sometimes at a distant site. The present consensus is that prophylactic radiation should remain the standard treatment, but current trials are assessing whether the area treated can be less extensive.

About 20% of patients with seminoma prove to have metastatic disease confined to the abdomen. Those with low volume (less than 5 cm, stages IIa and IIb) disease are conventionally treated with radiotherapy. Although rates of relapse for such patients will be higher than for those with stage I disease, cure rates remain high.[17] Several groups are investigating treatment of these patients with chemotherapy (such as carboplatin), though this must be regarded as experimental at present.

Patients with more bulky disease, those relapsing after radio-

37

therapy, and those with widespread disease at presentation are treated with chemotherapy. These patients, who are a minority, remain curable in at least 75% of cases. Current trials seek to determine the best chemotherapy regimen—the Medical Research Council is at present comparing a well tolerated treatment (single agent carboplatin)[18] with a more toxic combination of cisplatin and etoposide. At completion of treatment residual masses at the site of previous disease are common. These are probably best watched as most are benign and stabilise or resolve; surgery is difficult in this situation and residual cancer comparatively rare.

Other germ cell tumours

Mediastinal and pineal germ cell tumours

Mediastinal germ cell tumours occur almost exclusively in men and pineal and suprasellar germ cell tumours in children of both sexes. Histologically these tumours mimic their testicular counterparts and both pure seminoma (known as germinoma in the central nervous system) and malignant teratoma are well described; yolk sac tumours are particularly common in the mediastinum.[19]

Mediastinal germ cell tumours are often far advanced at presentation (fig 4). Though seminoma is curable with chemotherapy[2] or, for small lesions, radiotherapy, the malignant teratomas are more refractory to treatment and cure rates are lower. High dose chemotherapy is usually used together with surgery in most cases. These tumours are associated with Klinefelter's syndrome and also with various haematological abnormalities[20]—for example, simultaneous pre-sentation of teratoma and acute myeloid leukaemia is well described.

Pineal germinomas can be cured with radiotherapy.[21] Pineal or suprasellar teratomas (diagnosed either by biopsy or raised α fetoprotein concentrations in the blood or cerebrospinal fluid) should be managed with chemotherapy with a substantial chance of cure.[22]

Ovarian germ cell tumours

Ovarian seminoma (usually known as dysgerminoma) and teratoma are much less common than testicular germ cell tumours but occur in a comparably young population. These cancers can be managed in a similar fashion with a high expectation of cure—that is, combination chemotherapy containing cisplatin for metastatic disease and a watch

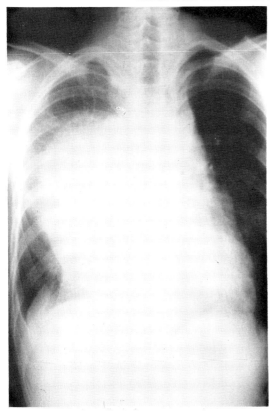

Figure 4—Huge anterior mediastinal mass at presentation in 21 year old. No biopsy was done before treatment; his α fetoprotein concentration of 114 000 U/l was diagnostic of mediastinal teratoma

policy (or radiation for dysgerminoma) for patients with stage I disease.[23]

Follow up

Most patients with widespread germ cell cancers who achieve a complete remission remain disease free. Long term sequelae of treatment are relatively slight, fertility is often preserved, and a return to normal employment is usual.[24] Early relapse carries a relatively poor prognosis, though new high dose treatments may cure even patients who have been heavily treated.[25] Late relapse occurs in a small percentage of cases and often carries a much better prognosis.

Conclusion

The most remarkable advance in therapeutic oncology during the past 10-15 years has been in the treatment of germ cell tumours. A high proportion of patients with these cancers are now entered into large cooperative clinical trials, which hold the key to improvements in management in the future. These tumours are diverse and their management complex; referral to specialist oncology centres with the wide range of expertise necessary to treat these fascinating neoplasms should be considered in all cases.

1 Senturia YD. The epidemiology of testicular cancer. *Br J Urol* 1987;**60**: 285-91
2 Loehrer PJ Sr, Williams SD, Einhorn LH. Testicular cancer: the quest continues. *J Natl Cancer Inst* 1988;**80**:1373-82.
3 Reinbery Y, Manivel JC, Fraley EE. Carcinoma in situ of the testis. *J Urol* 1989;**142**:243-7.
4 Von der Maase H, Rørth M, Walbom-Jørgensen S, Sørensen BL, Christopherson IS, Hald T, *et al.* Carcinoma in situ of contralateral testis in patients with testicular germ cell cancer: study of 27 cases in 500 patients. *BMJ* 1986;**293**:1398-401.
5 Read G, Stenning SP, Cullen MH, Parkinson MC, Horwich A, Kaye SB, *et al.* Medical Research Council prospective study of surveillance for stage I testicular teratoma. *J Clin Oncol* (in press).
6 Freedman LS, Parkinson MC, Jones WG, Oliver RTD, Peckham MJ, Read G, *et al.* Histopathology in the prediction of relapse of patients with stage I testicular teratoma treated by orchidectomy alone. *Lancet* 1987;ii: 294-8
7 McKendrick JJ, Theaker J, Mead GM. Non seminomatous germ cell tumour (NSGCT) with very high serum human chorionic gonadotrophin. *Cancer* 1991;**67**:684-9.
8 Mead GM, Stenning SP, Parkinson MC, Horwich A, Fossa SD, Wilkinson PM, *et al.* The second Medical Research Council study of prognostic factors in non-seminomatous germ cell tumours. *J Clin Oncol* 1992;**10**: 85-94.
9 Jansen RLH, Sylvester R, Sleyfer DT, ten Bokkel Huinink WW, Kaye SB, Jones WG, *et al.* Long-term follow up of non-seminomatous testicular cancer patients with mature teratoma or carcinoma at postchemotherapy surgery. *Eur J Cancer* 1991;**27**:695.
10 Dearnaley DP, Horwich A, A'Hern R, Nicholls J, Jay G, Hendry WF, *et al.* Combination chemotherapy with bleomycin, etoposide, and cisplatin (BEP) for metastatic testicular teratoma: long term follow up. *Eur J Cancer* 1991;**27**:684-91.
11 Einhorn LH, Williams SD, Loehrer PJ, Birch R, Drasga R, Omura G, *et al.* Evaluation of optimal duration of chemotherapy in favourable-prognosis disseminated germ cell tumours: a Southeastern Cancer Study Group protocol. *J Clin Oncol* 1989;**7**:387-91.
12 Horwich A, Dearnaley DP, Nicholls J, Jay G, Mason M, Harland S, *et al.* Effectiveness of carboplatin, etoposide, and bleomycin combination chemotherapy in good-prognosis metastatic testicular nonseminomatous germ cell tumours. *J Clin Oncol* 1991;**9**:62-9.
13 Nichols CR, Williams SD, Loehrer PJ, Greco FA, Crawford ED, Weetlaufer J, *et al.* Randomised study of cisplatin dose intensity in poor-risk germ cell tumours: a Southeastern Cancer Study Group and Southwest Oncology Group protocol. *J Clin Oncol* 1991;**7**:1163-72.
14 Lewis CR, Fossa SD, Mead G, ten Bokkel Huinink W, Harding MJ, Mill L, *et al.* BOP/VIP— a new platinum-intensive chemotherapy regimen for poor prognosis germ cell tumours. *Ann Oncol* 1991;**2**:203-11.
15 Fossa SD, Aass N, Kaalhus O. Radiotherapy for testicular seminoma stage I: treatment results and long-term post-irradiation morbidity in 365 patients. *Int J Rad Oncol Biol Phys* 1989;**16**:383-8.
16 Duchesne GM, Horwich A, Dearnaley DP, Nicholls J, Peckham MJ, Hendry WF, *et al.* Orchidectomy alone for stage I seminoma of the testis. *Cancer* 1990;**65**:1115-8.
17 Gregory C, Peckham MJ. Results of radiotherapy for stage II testicular seminoma. *Radiother Oncol* 1986;**6**:285-92.

18 Horwich A, Dearnaley DP, Duchesne GM, Williams M, Brada M, Peckham MJ. Simple nontoxic treatment of advanced metastatic seminoma with carboplatin. *J Clin Oncol* 1989;**7**:1150-6.

19 Nichols GR, Saxman S, Williams D, Löehrer PJ, Miller ME, Wright C, *et al*. Primary mediastinal nonseminomatous germ cell tumours. A modern single institution experience. *Cancer* 1990;**65**:1641-6.

20 Nichols GR, Roth BJ, Hefrema N, Griep J, Tricot G, *et al*. Hematologic neoplasia associated with primary mediastinal germ-cell tumors. *N Engl J Med* 1990;**322**:1425-9.

21 Dearnaley DP, A'Hern RP, Whittacker S, Bloom HJG. Pineal and CNS germ cell tumours: Royal Marsden Hospital experience 1962-1987. *Int J Rad Oncol Biol Phys* 1990;**10**:773-81.

22 Smith DB, Newlands ES, Begent RHJ, Rustin GSJ, Bagshawe KD. Optimum management of pineal germ cell tumours. *Clin Oncol* 1991;**3**:96-9.

23 Gershenson DM, Morris M, Cangir A, Kayanagh JJ, Stringer CA, Edwards CL, *et al*. Treatment of malignant germ cell tumours of the ovary with bleomycin, etoposide and cisplatin. *J Clin Oncol* 1990;**8**:715-20.

24 Roth BJ, Greist A, Kubilis PS, Williams SD, Einhorm LH. Cisplatin-based combination chemotherapy for disseminated germ cell tumours: long-term follow up. *J Clin Oncol* 1988;**6**:1239-47.

25 Nichols CR, Tricot G, Williams SD, van Besien K, Loehrer PJ, Roth BJ, *et al*. Dose-intensive chemotherapy in refractory germ cell cancer—a phase I/II trial of high-dose carboplatin and etoposide with autologous bone marrow transplantation. *J Clin Oncol* 1989;**7**:932-9.

Ovarian and cervical cancer

CHRIS WILLIAMS

Ovarian carcinoma

Ovarian carcinoma has been increasing in incidence and it is now the commonest malignancy of the female genital tract in most of the Western world. About 4500 women in England and Wales develop this cancer each year and there are 3700 deaths annually. The death rate of 14/100 000 has doubled in the past 70 years even when standardised for age. Incidences for this tumour are low in Asia, Africa, and South America and are, in any individual country, higher in the professional classes. Despite these data suggesting environmental factors in its causation, little is known about such factors.

Risk of ovarian cancer is reduced by pregnancy and is highest in infertile women. Use of oral contraceptives also reduces the risk, though this may partly reflect the increased risk in infertile women. The lowest risk is, curiously, seen in women who have had tubal ligation. There is also a reduction in risk among women who have had a hysterectomy but whose ovaries were conserved. Despite this there has been a vigorous debate in the United States about whether women approaching the menopause who are undergoing a hysterectomy should also have a bilateral oophorectomy.[1]

Up to 5% of women who develop ovarian carcinoma have a strong family history of this tumour, and many of these families may have a genetic predisposition to developing ovarian, and sometimes other, cancers.[2 3] Inheritance is probably autosomal dominant and researchers are close to identifying the gene(s) involved.

42

Diagnosis and surgery

Screening for ovarian cancer has been evaluated extensively in pilot studies. Although transvaginal ultrasonography with or without colour Doppler and screening for CA 125 have been shown capable of detecting "early" ovarian carcinoma, specificity remains an important problem.[4] So far no studies have shown that early detection of ovarian cancer by screening improves survival, and its general use cannot be recommended. The United Kingdom Coordinating Committee for Cancer Research has proposed a national study of familial ovarian cancer, and this will offer screening to high risk family members.

Most patients with ovarian cancer have had non-specific symptoms for some weeks or for a few months before diagnosis. Patients rarely present as surgical emergencies. So there is time to investigate and plan surgery before undertaking a laparotomy. This is important as surgery seems to be a keystone to prolonged survival.[5] As well as carrying out thorough staging, current surgical recommendations include, where appropriate, an attempt at maximum debulking (residual tumour masses <1·5 cm diameter) when complete clearance of tumours is not possible. This flies in the face of usual surgical tenets and surgeons not used to dealing with this tumour may fail to debulk even when this is possible. Despite lack of properly controlled trials testing the effectiveness of debulking surgery, current consensus suggests that debulked tumours are more responsive to chemotherapy and that patients with such tumours may survive longer and have better quality of life (fig 1).[6] The development of chemotherapy

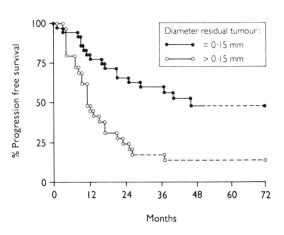

Figure 1—Relation between disease free survival after combination chemotherapy and diameter of largest tumour mass after primary cytoreductive surgery.[6] (Reproduced by permission of "Gynecologic Oncology," Academic Press)

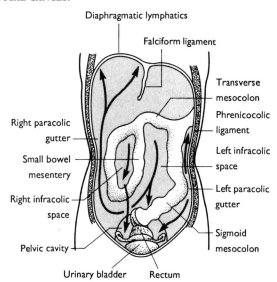

Diaphragmatic lymphatics

Falciform ligament

Transverse mesocolon

Phrenicocolic ligament

Left infracolic space

Left paracolic gutter

Sigmoid mesocolon

Right paracolic gutter

Small bowel mesentery

Right infracolic space

Pelvic cavity

Urinary bladder   Rectum

Figure 2 — Circulation of peritoneal fluid within the abdominal cavity. (Reproduced by permission of Chapman and Hall)

capable of curing advanced disease is, however, likely to render surgical debulking obsolete.

Radiotherapy

There is little evidence that radiotherapy has any role in managing ovarian cancer in women who have not had maximum debulking surgery or complete excision of the tumour. Thus any potential benefit may be in patients with "early stage" disease who have had optimal surgery. Even in these women there is debate about its effectiveness.

Studies into mechanisms of tumour spread (fig 2)[7] and staging in the past two decades have clearly shown that the whole of the abdominal cavity is at risk of relapse in such women so pelvic irradiation alone is likely to prove inadequate. Unfortunately, only modest radiation doses can be delivered to the whole abdominal contents (2250 cGy in 30 fractions over four to six weeks, for example). And such doses may be inadequate to eliminate even microscopic metastases. Nevertheless, a series of randomised trials from Toronto have strongly suggested improved survival in women with stage I-III ovarian carcinoma undergoing optimal surgery who were treated with whole abdominal radiation compared with pelvic radiation with or without an alkylating drug.[8] Similar randomised studies at the M D Anderson

TABLE I—Five year survival by stage in collected series of patients with ovarian carcinoma[10]

	No (%) of cases	% Alive at 5 years
Stage I	2449 (24)	67
Stage II	1806 (19)	42
Stage III and IV	5540 (57)	14·4

Hospital, however, have not supported these results.[9] Smaller studies have also failed to show benefit for radiation. Currently, radiation is being little studied and is not used routinely by many centres. There may well still be a place, however, for well designed large trials testing its use as an adjuvant to surgery.

Chemotherapy

Ovarian cancer was one of the first tumours to be routinely treated with chemotherapy. Alkylating drugs rapidly became a standard treatment for advanced ovarian cancer and it is on these patients, the majority (table I), that most data are available. Numerous randomised clinical trials have tested the effectiveness of different types of chemotherapy in stage III and IV disease but there are few data comparing chemotherapy with a no treatment control. These studies have all been of modest size (50-300 patients) and it is therefore unsurprising that nearly all have failed to show significant differences between the treatments being tested. Despite this therapeutic fashions have evolved and changed over the past 15 years (box).

Because of the lack of reliable data the Medical Research Council in Britain organised a systematic overview of chemotherapy for advanced ovarian malignancy. This exhaustive meta-analysis of all the individual patient data from properly randomised trials, published and unpublished, comparing single drugs with combinations and assessing the role of platinum has recently been published.[11]

Despite including over 8000 patients with advanced disease, of whom more than 6500 had died, this overview did not provide clear guidance about the best available current therapy. Rather it has defined questions suitable for large trials. Although little evidence exists that platinum prolongs survival when compared with an oral alkylating drug, platinum therapy is generally considered to be the first choice. This is based on its undoubtedly higher objective

Therapeutic fashions in chemotherapy of advanced ovarian carcinoma

Before 1976   Single oral alkylating agent such as chlorambucil.

↓

1976   Non-cisplatin based combination such as HEXACAF (hexamethylmelamine, cyclophosphamide, methotrexate, fluorouracil)

↓

1980   Cisplatin based combination such as CAP (cyclophosphamide, doxorubicin, cisplatin)

↓

1985   Removal of doxorubicin from CAP type combinations, leaving cyclophosphamide and cisplatin

↓

1988   Treatment with single agent cisplatin

↓

1990   Substitution of carboplatin for cisplatin

↓

1991   Overview suggests superiority of CAP over cisplatin alone. Further studies started.

response rate, the likely consequent better control of symptoms, and the fact that many patients initially treated with an alkylating drug subsequently receive platinum on disease progression or relapse. Based on this, the finding that carboplatin is equally effective as cisplatin, and the suggestion that the addition of other drugs to platinum improves survival (fig 3),[11] a large scale trial for advanced ovarian carcinoma has begun. This study, sponsored by the Medical Research Council, compares a relatively non-toxic treatment, carboplatin, with cisplatin, doxorubicin, and cyclophosphamide (CAP) to test whether there is a survival advantage for the more toxic combination.

Since the trials of adjuvant chemotherapy for "early" disease are too small a parallel trial is comparing immediate platinum based chemotherapy with chemotherapy given at relapse. Both trials are being conducted by the International Collaborative Ovarian Neoplasm (ICON) Group. They are both international and the aim is to accrue 2000 patients in each trial.

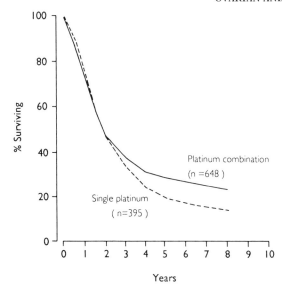

Figure 3 — Survival of patients treated with single agent platinum and platinum combinations. Imbalance in patient numbers is caused by randomised trials comparing single agent platinum with two combinations

Summary

The incidence of ovarian cancer continues to increase steadily and it now accounts for 1·3% of all deaths in women or 6% of deaths from cancer in women. No convincing aetiological factor has been identified. Debate still surrounds the concept of oophorectomy at the time of hysterectomy and an appropriately controlled trial is needed. Familial ovarian cancer may account for up to 5% of cases, and the gene(s) may soon be identified. Screening can be considered in family members but general population screening cannot be recommended.

Radiotherapy is used rarely. When employed whole abdominal fields should be used after removal of all or most of the tumour. The best chemotherapy regimen remains undefined despite numerous small trials. Platinum drugs are generally accepted as the most active group of drugs and adding other drugs may further improve survival. This hypothesis is being tested in the first large scale study of chemotherapy in ovarian carcinoma.

Carcinoma of the cervix

Invasive carcinoma of the cervix is the sixth commonest cancer in British women, with an annual incidence of 16/100000 women. It accounts for about 4% of female malignancy and has a five year survival of 58%, which is better than many other common cancers. Despite this there is a real need for improvement in its management.

About 90% of invasive cervical tumours are squamous carcinomas, which usually arise from the squamo-columnar junction. The remainder are generally adenocarcinomas, arising from the endocervical glands in the endocervical mucosa, or mixed squamous adenocarcinomas. Since many tumours seem to have arisen after the initial development of a precursor premalignant condition (cervical intraepithelial neoplasia) screening for these lesions has been a cornerstone of attempts to reduce mortality.

The death rate from cervical cancer has fallen sharply in many developed countries: a phenomenon often explained by the introduction of screening, though this fall preceded the introduction of screening in many countries. Unfortunately, there were no randomised trials of cervical screening when it was first introduced so its contribution to falling mortality rates can be only guessed at. Despite this most workers in the subject support its use and the recent strategy document from the Department of Health, *The Health of the Nation*, included targets for cervical cancer screening.

Unfortunately, the target is only that all women aged 20-64 years be invited for screening by the end of 1993. This fails to overcome some of the problems associated with the cervical smear programme. The most important of these is that women at greatest risk of cervical cancer are the ones most likely to fail to accept an invitation for screening. At present 60% of women who develop cervical cancer have never been screened. Although general practitioners have been asked to fulfil screening targets in return for financial reward, inner city practices, where the incidence is highest, may see these targets as non-achievable and consequently be deterred from making a big effort. Help is needed in devising strategies which encourage women at risk to attend for screening.

A second problem is the adequacy of smears that are taken—any targets set should specify the rate of smears which are considered to be adequate for reporting.[12] Inadequate smears cause anxiety for patients recalled, discourage future screening, and add to an already not inconsiderable cost. Changes in technique (Aylesbury spatula and cytobrush, for instance) and improved technical competence should reduce rates of inadequate smears to about 5%. Interpretation of cervical smears requires a high degree of skill, and audit systems should be mandatory in cytology units. However, even in the best laboratories the false negative rate may be as high as 10%.[12]

Because most cervical intraepithelial neoplasias evolve into invasive tumours only very slowly many clinicians have believed that follow up investigation of such lesions is not especially urgent. Because of pressure on colposcopy and other resources women in Britain often wait months before further investigation after an abnormal smear test result. This is unacceptable, not least because of the anxiety caused by such a delay but also because of the risk that there is already an invasive tumour—cytology may not detect concomitant invasive carcinomas. A prerequisite of any screening system is that a highly efficient mechanism is already in place to deal with women with positive screening test results. Cervical carcinoma fulfils most of the potential requirements for a successful screening programme—it remains to be seen whether there is the will to make it work. This means that any cervical screening programme must address the specific concerns of the women being screened, especially those at greatest risk.

Management of cervical intraepithelial neoplasia

There remains much debate about the best way to care for women with cervical intraepithelial neoplasia.[13] At least 50% of women with advanced lesions (grade III—severe dysplasia or carcinoma in situ) will go on to develop an invasive cancer if left untreated. In women with lower grade lesions (grades I and II) the rate of development of subsequent invasive cancer is lower. At present patients likely to progress to invasive tumour cannot be reliably detected, so ideally, from the point of view of preventing an invasive tumour, all patients should be referred for further investigation and treatment. This has enormous resource implications and also causes stress and anxiety to the patients, many of whom may not have gone on to develop an invasive carcinoma.

Cytology may be the best way of detecting cervical intraepithelial neoplasia but is not adequate for its evaluation. Most centres in Britain use colposcopy for evaluating neoplasia and for deciding on suitability of treatment with ablative procedures such as cryosurgery, laser, diathermy, cold coagulation, or cone biopsy. Ablation is successful in at least 80% of women, but those having an abnormal smear test result after ablation have a 25-fold increased risk of developing an invasive tumour. Further treatment will need to be planned, taking into account younger women's reproductive desires;

TABLE II—Randomised clinical trials producing five year survival data for management of operable cervical carcinoma (stages Ib, IIa)

Trial	Stage	No of patients	5 Year survival (%)	
			Radiation	Surgery
Cullhed[11]	Ib, IIa	310	75	86
Morley and Seski[15]	I	401	83	87
Newton[16]	I	119	74	81
Perez[17]	I	78	88	82
	IIa	24	71	57

older women may find the alternative to further ablation, hysterectomy, more acceptable. Thorough discussion of the pros and cons is needed—repeated ablation carries its own risks, including cervical stenosis and failure to prevent an invasive tumour developing. Long term follow up is mandatory in all cases.

Treatment of invasive cancer

Early invasive cervical carcinoma (stage Ib and IIa, table II) is treated equally well by radical hysterectomy or radiotherapy, though the pattern of side effects varies.[18 19] For more advanced disease (stages IIb-IVa) radiotherapy is generally the best treatment, though some centres will also undertake surgery in selected patients after irradiation. Many patients are treated with intracavitary radioactive isotopes, which deliver a very high dose to the central pelvis. The isotope is inserted under general anaesthesia, and the recent introduction of remote afterloading machines has considerably reduced treatment times and exposure of staff to radiation. Further external beam radiotherapy is usually given to treat the pelvic lymph nodes.

Success rates decrease with increasing tumour bulk and stage (table III). Very advanced or recurrent disease, which is not treatable by irradiation, and previously irradiated tumours have been managed recently by combinations of cytotoxic drugs based on cisplatin. Though such treatment is not curative, high objective response rates (50-60%) have been reported.[21] Because of this some units have tried using chemotherapy as part of the primary management. So far it is not clear if this approach of adjuvant chemotherapy will prolong survival of patients with cervical cancer, as has been shown in premenopausal women with breast cancer.[22] Most researchers using this approach have given chemotherapy before irradiation in an

TABLE III—Carcinoma of cervix: survival by stage of disease (results for 1969-72)[20]

	No of patients treated	No (%) surviving at 5 years
Stage I	12 452	9 961 (80·0)
Stage II	13 583	8 005 (58·9)
Stage III	10 531	3 287 (31·2)
Stage IV	1 841	153 (8·3)
Not staged	54	24 (44·4)
Total	38 461	21 430 (55·7)

attempt to shrink the tumour and to eradicate microscopic metastases.

Randomised trials testing adjuvant chemotherapy have been small and past experience, primarily in the adjuvant treatment of breast cancer, has clearly shown that large numbers of patients are needed before the success or otherwise of adjuvant treatment can be judged. The Medical Research Council is coordinating a series of randomised clinical trials testing the role of chemotherapy before irradiation or surgery, or both (so called neoadjuvant treatment) in patients with cervical carcinoma who are considered to be at risk of relapse based on tumour bulk or stage. The council is also gathering data from similar trials taking place worldwide to undertake a prospective meta-analysis. Until there are data to show that it improves survival adjuvant chemotherapy for cervical cancer should be regarded as experimental.

Summary

Death rates from cervical cancer have already fallen this century, and for patients with invasive cervical cancer five year survival rates are greater than for most solid tumours. Better screening for premalignant changes may further reduce the incidence of invasive cancer; indeed, it has been claimed that the reduction in mortality could be as high as 90%, though estimates of screening efficacy have varied greatly. For those with advanced invasive carcinoma neo-adjuvant chemotherapy may reduce the risk of relapse and improve survival.

1 Mack TM, Cozen W, Quinn MA. Epidemiology of cancer of the endometrium, ovary, and vagina. In: Coppleson M, ed. *Gynecologic oncology.* New York: Churchill Livingstone, 1992.

2 Lynch HT, Bewtra C, Lynch JF. Familial ovarian carcinoma. Clinical nuances. *Am J Med* 1986;**81**:1073-6.
3 Ponder BA. Genetic predisposition to cancer. *Br J Cancer* 1991;**64**:203-4.
4 Cuckle HS, Wald NJ. The evaluation of screening tests for ovarian cancer. In: *Ovarian cancer: biological and therapeutic challenges*. London: Chapman and Hall Medical, 1990:229-39.
5 Richardson GS, Scully RE, Ni N, Nelson JH. Common epithelial cancer of the ovary. *N Engl J Med* 1985;**312**:415-24.
6 Heintz AP, Van Oosterom AT, Trimbos JB, Schaberg A, Van der Velde E, Nooy M. The treatment of ovarian carcinoma. I. Clinical variables associated with prognosis. *Gynecol Oncol* 1988;**30**:347-58.
7 Pickel. Intraperitoneal and retroperitoneal spread of ovarian cancer In: Sharp F, Mason W, Leake R, eds. *Ovarian cancer: biological and therapeutic challenges*. London: Chapman and Hall, 1990.
8 Dembo AJ, Bush RS, Beale F, Bean H, Pringle J, Sturgeon J. The Princess Margaret Hospital study of ovarian cancer: stage I, II and asymptomatic III presentations. *Cancer Treatment Reports* 1979;**63**:249-56.
9 Smith JP, Rutledge FN, Declos L. Postoperative treatment of early cancer of the ovary: a random trial between post operative irradiation and chemotherapy. *National Cancer Institute Monograms* 1975;**42**:149-53.
10 Morrow CP. In: Coppleson M, ed. *Gynecologic oncology*. New York: Churchill Livingstone, 1992:897.
11 Advanced Ovarian Cancer Trialists Group. Chemotherapy in advanced ovarian cancer: an overview of randomised clinical trials. *BMJ* 1991;**303**: 884-93.
12 Ng ABP. Diagnostic cytopathology. In: Coppleson M, ed. *Gynecologic oncology*. New York: Churchill Livingstone, 1992:277-96.
13 Coppleson M, Atkinson KH, Dalrymple JC. Cervical squamous and glandular intraepithelial neoplasm: clinical features and review of management. In: Coppleson M, ed. *Gynecologic oncology*. New York: Churchill Livingstone, 1992:571-607.
14 Cullhed S. Carcinoma cervicis uteri stages I and IIa. *Acta Obstet Gynecol Scand* 1978;suppl **78**: 1-149
15 Morley G, Seski J. Radical pelvic surgery versus radiation therapy for stage I carcinoma of the cervix (exclusive of microinvasion). *Am J Obstet Gynecol* 1976;**126**:785-96
16 Newton M. Radical hysterectomy or radiotherapy for stage I cervical cancer. A prospective comparison with 5 and 10 years follow-up. *Am J Obstet Gynecol* 1975;**123**:534-42.
17 Perez CA, Camel HM, Kao MS, Askin F. Randomised study of preoperative radiation and surgery or irradiation alone in treatment of stage Ib and IIa carcinoma of the uterine cervix. *Cancer* 1980;**45**:2759-68.
18 Averett HE, La Platney DR, Little WA. Current role of radical hysterectomy as primary therapy for invasive carcinoma of the cervix. *Am J Obstet Gynecol* 1969;**105**:79-86.
19 Jampolis S, Andras J, Fletcher GH. Analysis of sites and causes of failure of irradiation in invasive squamous cell carcinoma of the intact uterine cervix. *Radiology* 1975;**115**:681-5.
20 International Federation of Gynaecology and Obstetrics. *Seventeenth annual report. Radiumhemmet Stockholm: IFGO, 1977.*
21 Buxton EJ, Meanwell CA, Hilton C, Mould JJ, Spooner D, Chetiyawardona A, *et al*. Combination bleomycin, ifosfamide, and cisplatin chemotherapy in cervical cancer. *J Natl Cancer Inst* 1989;**81**:359-61.
22 Early Breast Cancer Trialists Collaborative Group. Systemic treatment of early breast cancer by hormonal, cytotoxic, or immune therapy. *Lancet* 1992; **339**:1-14, 71-84.

Colorectal cancer

R H J BEGENT

Each year 22 000 people die of cancer of the colon and rectum in Britain, making this disease the second most common cause of death from cancer. Five year survival is less than 30%, and until recently surgery was the only treatment that reduced mortality. Moves are now being made towards more screening, adjuvant therapy, and intensive follow up with resection or chemotherapy for recurrence. Implementation of these policies requires structured planning rather than reaction to crises.

These trends have stronger support in the United States than in Britain, where there has been concern that quality of life will be diminished by introducing unproved investigation or treatment. Validated methods of measurement of quality of life make it possible to address such concerns.[1] This chapter considers the case for a more prospective and active approach to management of colorectal cancer. The various stages of management are listed in table I.

TABLE I—Components of management of colorectal cancer

Component	Requirements or comments
Case finding	Public and professional awareness
Screening	Family history, genetic markers, knowledge of predisposing conditions
Surgical resection	Specialist colorectal surgeons
Adjuvant therapy	Some indications but more trials needed
Follow up	Role of intensive follow up uncertain
Palliation	Chemotherapy and radiotherapy useful; quality of life must be assessed

Screening

Sigmoidoscopy

The benefits of sigmoidoscopy in healthly populations are contro-versial. The proposal that sigmoidoscopy, preferably with a flexibile instrument, should be done every three to five years in people over the age of 50 is supported by the National Cancer Institute of the United States, the American Cancer Society, and the American College of Physicians. However, the King's Fund consensus statement,[2] the United States preventive services task force, and the Canadian periodic health examination task force considered that the case for screening was not strong enough. A casecontrol study has since shown a 59% reduction in mortality from bowel cancer in people screened by sigmoidoscopy, with the reduction applying only to tumours arising in the screened part of the bowel.[3]

The potential benefit of screening comes largely from identifying and removing premalignant adenomas, though carcinomas may also be diagnosed. Evidence that sigmoidoscopy rather than colonoscopy is appropriate for initial screening comes from a study in which the standardised incidence ratio of colonic cancer was 3·6 if a single villous, tubulovillous, or large (>1 cm) adenoma was found in the rectosigmoid by rigid sigmoidoscopy.[4] If the adenomas were multiple the standardised incidence ratio was 6·6. Thus a large, tubulovillous, or villous adenoma in the rectosigmoid seems to be predictive of carcinoma at remote proximal sites in the colon and such patients should have follow up by colonoscopy. The case for routine screening of people aged over 50 by sigmoidoscopy should be re-examined.

Faecal occult blood

Large randomised studies of the value of faecal occult blood testing in healthy populations are in progress, but definitive results in terms of mortality cannot be expected until 1995. Sensitivity and specificity are limited but a higher proportion of good prognosis (Dukes's stage A) tumours is detected in screened populations than in controls.[5]

High risk groups

Family doctors, surgeons, and clinical oncologists have an import-ant role in identifying risk by taking a comprehensive family history and acting on it. Right sided tumours, carcinoma occurring at a young age, familial adenomatous polyposis, a carcinoma in a first degree relative, and family history of ovarian, breast, or uterine carcinoma,

54

particularly at a young age, are pointers to a possible familial risk. Assessment of risk by a clinical geneticist is particularly valuable in such cases and the development of genetic markers—for example, in familial adenomatous polyposis—is increasing the precision of risk assessment. Colonoscopy should be done regularly in these people[6] as well as in those with ulcerative colitis or who have had resection of a carcinoma or adenoma.

Intitial surgery

Operative mortality and postoperative morbidity and survival are better, especially for rectal cancer, if surgery is done by a specialist colorectal surgeon.[78] The King's Fund consensus statement on colorectal cancer considered that the evidence was strong enough to recommend that arrangements should be made in each British health district for a specialist emergency and elective service or for patients to be referred to a hospital that makes this provision.[2] This could be achieved if health authorities placing contracts for cancer care made it a required quality criterion.

Adjuvant therapy in rectal carcinoma

Rectal and colonic carcinoma are considered separately because local recurrence of rectal carcinoma in the pelvis gives radiotherapy a role in treatment of rectal carcinoma which does not apply to colonic tumours (table II).

Radiotherapy

Local recurrence occurs in about one third of patients after

TABLE II—Current recommendations for adjuvant therapy

Site and stage	Recommended adjuvant therapy
Rectum:	
A	None
B	Radiotherapy and chemotherapy
C	Radiotherapy and chemotherapy
Colon:	
A	None
B	None
C	Chemotherapy

apparently complete resection of rectal cancer and is more common when there is local infiltration into perirectal tissues or on to serosal surfaces. Radiotherapy either before or after surgery reduces this incidence. Preoperative treatment has lower morbidity, but patients with early disease and little chance of recurrence may be treated unnecessarily. Survival benefit from perioperative radiotherapy has not been shown conclusively, but combined analysis of the relevant trials suggests a benefit of about 10%. More data on survival are expected shortly from mature analysis of the Medical Research Council's second and third trials of radiotherapy, and the issue is being studied further in the United Kingdom Coordinating Committee on Cancer Research AXIS trial (Adjuvant X ray and Infusion Study).

Chemotherapy

Chemotherapy given in addition to postoperative radiotherapy prolongs survival in patients at high risk of recurrence. In a randomised study patients with nodal disease or infiltration through the muscle layers received radiation alone or radiation with chemotherapy.[9] 5-Fluorouracil was given with radiotherapy and 5-fluorouracil with semustine before and after radiotherapy. There was a significant reduction in the local recurrence rate in the group receiving chemotherapy in addition to radiotherapy, which was suggested to be the result of the radiosensitising effect of 5-fluorouracil given concurrently with radiotherapy. The overall death rate was reduced by 29% with the addition of chemotherapy. This study is the most convincing to date, but before its publication a consensus statement from the National Cancer Institute in the United States considered that there was strong evidence in favour of chemotherapy for Dukes's stage B and C carcinoma of the rectum.[10]

At present, inadequate information is available to recommend what the chemotherapy regimen should be. The trials needed to answer such questions require large numbers of patients and prolonged follow up. Several trials of different aspects of adjuvant chemotherapy and radiotherapy for rectal cancer are in progress and the most constructive approach is to enter patients into these. In Britain the AXIS trial addresses a relevant question in that patients are randomised to no chemotherapy or portal vein infusion of 5-fluorouracil for seven days after surgery. 5-Fluorouracil given in this way has access to the systemic circulation and could contribute to disease control in the

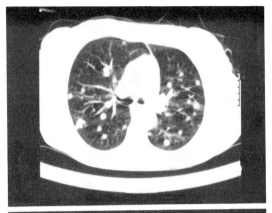

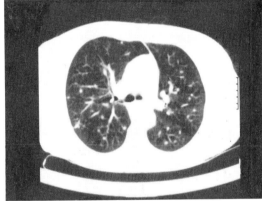

Computed tomograms showing (above) lung metastases before treatment and (below) after 12 weeks of chemotherapy with 5-fluorouracil and leucovorin

pelvis and elsewhere but is unlikely to have a radiosensitising effect, being given before radiotherapy.

Adjuvant therapy in colonic carcinoma

5-Fluorouracil gives partial or complete response in 10-15% of patients with advanced disease and the argument for using it as adjuvant treatment after apparently complete tumour resection is weak. Perhaps surprisingly, meta-analysis of trials of adjuvant therapy including 5-fluorouracil showed a small (3·4%) but significant survival benefit for treatment.[11] This has not in general been accepted as sufficient reason for using intravenous 5-fluorouracil for adjuvant therapy. Many trials combining 5-fluorouracil with other agents have given disappointing results.[12]

Developments incorporating 5-fluorouracil seem more interesting. Infusion of 5-fluorouracil into the portal vein for seven days after resection of the primary tumour gave impressive results in some trials.[13] Other trials have shown no benefit from this approach and it is being further investigated in the AXIS trial. The trial has the advantage that the treatment is completed during admission to hospital for primary surgery. Patients with all Dukes's stages are eligible but many surgeons prefer to omit patients with Dukes's stage A tumours because of their good survival without adjuvant therapy.

The combination of 5-fluorouracil and levamisole as adjuvant therapy has been shown to produce a significant survival advantage over levamisole alone and over no treatment in patients with Dukes's stage C colonic carcinoma.[14 15] The death rate was reduced by a third compared with controls. For patients with Dukes's stage B2 disease (tumour affecting pericolic fat or the serosa) a significant advantage in survival was not shown, but there were relatively few patients in this arm and longer follow up is needed before the case for adjuvant therapy in stage B disease can be judged. Levamisole, which was initially used for its antihelminthic properties, also has immuno-modulatory actions. Objectors to the adoption of this regimen point out that there was no 5-fluorouracil only arm in the major trial, although there was in a smaller study,[16] and that the place of levamisole as a single agent is not secure.[17]

5-Fluorouracil modulated by leucovorin has about double the response rate of 5-fluorouracil alone in patients with advanced disease. It is now being studied in randomised adjuvant therapy trials and results can be expected in the next few years. Until optimal chemotherapy regimens are established the best option is to enter patients into relevant clinical trials.

Follow up after initial treatment

Five year survival has changed little for colonic and rectal carcinoma in recent years. It is about 80% for Dukes's stage A, 50% for stage B, and 30% for stage C. Very few patients presenting with distant metastases or unresectable disease live for five years.

As many as 20% of patients relapsing after apparently curative resection can be cured by resection of hepatic or pulmonary metastases.[18] Results are best when there is a solitary deposit.

Intensive follow up can detect recurrence before it produces symptoms. Monthly measurements of serum carcinoembryonic antigen concentration predict clinically evident recurrence by an average of six months in about 60% of patients and trigger other investigations or exploratory laparotomy.[19] Other serum tumour markers may also contribute. Routine chest radiography, liver ultrasonography, and abdominal computed tomography and colonoscopy have also been used for early detection. Immunoscintigraphy can be helpful in locating metastases when serum carcinoembryonic antigen concentrations rise.[20]

As only solitary metastases will be curable and these will eventually be evident by simple clinical follow up and still be resectable, some people have argued against intensive follow up. In a randomised trial supported by the Cancer Research Campaign, serum carcinoembryonic antigen concentrations are measured regularly for three years. If there is a significant rise in antigen concentration patients are randomised to second look laparotomy and tumour resection unless there is a contraindication. In the control arm the surgeon is not informed of the antigen concentration and continues to follow up the patient in the normal way. Over 1100 patients have been entered but a result is not yet available.

Chemotherapy for advanced disease

Most tumour recurrences detected on follow up are not resectable, but could early diagnosis be beneficial in their management? The low response rate to 5-fluorouracil has rightly limited its use to palliation, but the higher response rates now achieved with combination therapy justify re-examination of this issue. A study in the Nordic countries randomised 183 patients with advanced but asymptomatic colorectal cancer for treatment either immediately or only when symptoms developed.[21] Median survival was five months longer (p<0·01) and the symptom free period six months longer (p<0·001) in patients treated with methotrexate, leucovorin, and 5-fluorouracil from the detection of their metastases rather than when symptoms developed. In a subset of patients in whom quality of life was assessed, those in the early treatment arm also fared better. If reproducible, this study argues for careful follow up including measurement of serum carcinoembryonic antigen concentration to give chemotherapy as soon as recurrence is detected.

59

Palliation

Radiotherapy is effective in palliation of symptoms produced by localised tumours, particularly in the pelvis. Chemotherapy also has a place in palliation.[2] Response rates with 5-fluorouracil alone are low (10-15%). The effect is dose related and infusion over a few days increases response rates.[22] The effect of 5-fluorouracil is modulated by administration with leucovorin, which prolongs the inhibition of thymidylate synthase activity and hence inhibits DNA synthesis through stabilisation of the ternary complex of 5,10-methylenetetrahydrofolic acid with fluorodeoxyuridine monophosphate (a metabolite of 5-fluorouracil) and thymidylate synthase. Response rates are increased to 20-40% and relief of symptoms is reported in up to 75% of patients. Increased survival compared with that after 5-fluorouracil alone has been reported.[23] Meta-analysis has not confirmed this report, although response rates were increased from 11% to 23% ($p < 10^{-7}$) with 5-fluorouracil and leucovorin compared with 5-fluorouracil alone.[24] The relatively low overall response rate and crossover of patients from one regimen to the other may conceal a survival benefit.

When metastases are confined to the liver 5-fluorodeoxyuridine infused through the hepatic artery produces higher response rates than intravenously administered 5-fluorouracil.[25] However, increased survival has not been shown, probably because of metastases outside the liver which were too small to detect when treatment was begun. A current trial of this approach is further investigating survival and quality of life.

These chemotherapy regimens are generally well tolerated but if there is no convincing survival benefit their use has to be justified by improved quality of life.[2] Data are sparse, but improved quality of life has been reported with one regimen of 5-fluorouracil and leucovorin compared with 5-fluorouracil alone.[22] More studies using validated quality of life assessments are necessary before the place of palliative chemotherapy can be properly assessed.

Future prospects

The outlook for people with colorectal cancer has improved slightly, and several new approaches being investigated in clinical trials may have a further impact.

Surgery

The frequency of local recurrence may be reduced by radio-immunoguided surgery. Antibodies reacting with colorectal cancer antigens and radiolabelled with iodine-125 are given intravenously before surgery and a hand held gamma detecting probe is used to locate the tumour at operation. Residual tumour, not detectable by conventional means, can be located in the tumour bed or at the margin of the resected specimen.[26] Occult metastases have also been detected.

Drug resistance

The best regimens containing 5-fluorouracil give only 20-40% response rates, and drug resistance eventually develops in almost all patients. The effects of 5-fluorouracil may be enhanced by modulation with drugs other than leucovorin. Interferon alfa is an example and is being studied in combination with 5-fluorouracil and leucovorin in a randomised trial. Uridine and dipyridamole are other modulators of pyrimidine metabolism whose roles are being investigated.

Biological therapy

New approaches based on our improved understanding of the molecular basis of neoplasia show promise. Clinical trials of antibody targeted therapy are in progress in colorectal cancer. Antibodies targeting colorectal cancer have been used to activate natural immune effector mechanisms, to target therapeutic radionuclides or toxins, and to target an enzyme which will activate a prodrug at the tumour site. A vaccine composed of a human antibody directed against the idiotype of an antitumour antibody mimics the tumour associated antigen but is immunogenic, breaking natural tolerance to the tumour antigen.

Conclusion

Surgery followed by only simple palliation for symptoms caused by advanced disease is no longer sufficient in management of colorectal cancer. Early diagnosis through case finding and screening of high risk groups can lead to treatment when prognosis is relatively good. Adjuvant chemotherapy and radiotherapy have a place but the best way of applying them is not clear and it is important that patients are entered into relevant clinical trials. Early chemotherapy for recurrence seems to improve survival, and if confirmed this would justify careful follow up after initial surgery. Particular attention should be paid to measuring quality of life in clinical trials and in routine practice. Teams including the relevant specialists are likely to be most effective in implementing these measures in an efficient and cost effective way.

I thank Dr J C Thompson for her help in preparing this article.

1 Byrne M. Cancer chemotherapy and quality of life. *BMJ* 1992;**304**:1523-4.
2 Seventh King's Fund Forum. *Cancer of the colon and rectum consensus statement.* London: King's Fund, 1990.
3 Selby JV, Friedman GD, Queensbury CP, Weiss NS. A case control study of screening sigmoidoscopy and mortality from colorectal cancer. *N Engl J Med* 1992;**326**:653-5.
4 Aitken WS, Morson BC, Cuzick J. Long term risk of colorectal cancer after excision of rectosigmoid adenomas. *N Engl J Med* 1992;**326**:658-62.
5 Hardcastle JD, Farrands PA, Balfour TW. Controlled trial of faecal occult blood testing in the detection of colorectal cancer. *Lancet* 1983;ii:1-4.
6 Houlston RS, Murday V, Harocopos C, Williams CB, Slack J. Screening and genetic counselling for relatives of patients with colorectal cancer in a family cancer clinic. *BMJ* 1990;**301**:18-25.
7 McArdle CS, Hole D. Impact of variability among surgeons on postoperative morbidity and mortality and ultimate survival. *BMJ* 1991;**302**:1501-5.
8 Darby CR, Berry AR, Mortensen N. Management variability in surgery for colorectal emergencies. *Br J Surg* 1992;**79**:206-10.
9 Krook JE, Moertel CG, Gunderson LL, Wieand LL, Collins RT, Beart RW, *et al.* Effective surgical adjuvant therapy of high risk rectal cancer. *N Engl J Med* 1991;**324**:709-45.
10 Office of Medical Applications of Research. NIH consensus conference. Adjuvant therapy for patients with colon and rectal cancer. *JAMA* 1990;**264**:1444-50.
11 Buyse M, Zeleniuch-Jacquotte A, Chambers TC. Adjuvant therapy of colorectal cancer. Why we still don't know. *JAMA* 1988;**259**:3571-8.
12 Schnall SF, MacDonald JS. Adjuvant therapy in colorectal cancer. *Semin Oncol* 1991;**18**: 560-70.
13 Taylor I, Machin D, Mullee M. A randomised controlled trial of adjuvant portal vein cytotoxic perfusion in colorectal cancer. *Br J Surg* 1985;**72**: 359-63.
14 Moertel CG, Fleming TR, MacDonald JS. Levamisole and fluorouracil in adjuvant therapy for resected colon cancer. *N Engl J Med* 1990;**322**: 352-8.
15 Moertel CG, Fleming T, Macdonald JS, Haller D, Laurie J. The intergroup study of fluorouracil (5-FU) plus levamisole (LEV) and levamisole alone as adjuvant therapy for stage C colon cancer. A final report (abstract). *Proceedings of the American Association of Clinical Oncology* 1992;May:457.
16 Windle R, Bell PRF, Shaw D. Five year results of a randomised trial of adjuvant 5-fluorouracil and levamisole in colorectal cancer. *Br J Surg* 1987;**74**:569-72.
17 Arnaud JP, Byse M, Nordlinger B. Adjuvant therapy of poor prognosis colon cancer with levamisole: results of an EORTC double blind randomised clinical trial. *Br J Surg* 1989;**76**:284-9.
18 August DA, Ottow RT, Sugarbaker PH. Clinical perspectives of human colorectal cancer metastases. *Cancer Metastasis Rev* 1984;**3**:303-24.
19 Begent RHJ, Rustin GJS. Tumour markers: from carcinoembryonic antigen to products of hybridoma technology. *Cancer Surv* 1989;**8**:108-21.
20 Begent RHJ, Keep PA, Searle F, Green AJ, Mitchell HDC, Jones BE, *et al.* Radioimmunolocalisation and selection for surgery in recurrent colorectal cancer. *Br J Surg* 1986;**73**:64-7.
21 Glimelius B for the Nordic Gastrointestinal Tumour Adjuvant Therapy Group. Expectancy of primary chemotherapy in paients with advanced asymptomatic colorectal cancer: a randomised trial. *Eur J Cancer* 1991; Suppl 2:S82.
22 Lokich JJ, Ahlgren JD, Gullo JJ, Phillips JA, Fryer JG. A prospective randomised comparison of continuous infusion fluorouracil with a conventional schedule in metastatic colorectal carcinoma. A mid-Atlantic oncology program study. *J Clin Oncol* 1989;**7**:425-32.

23 Poon MA, O'Connell MJ, Moertel CG, Wieand HS, Cullinan SA, Everson LK, *et al*. Biochemical modulation of fluorouracil: evidence of significant improvement of survival and quality of life in patients with advanced colorectal carcinoma. *J Clin Oncol* 1989;7:1407-18.

24 Piedbois P, Buyse M, Rustum Y, Machover D, Erlichman C, Carlson RW, *et al*. Modulation of 5-fluorouracil by leucovorin in patients with advanced colorectal cancer: a meta-analysis (abstract). *Proceedings of the American Society of Clinical Oncology* 1992;May:1026.

25 Chang AE, Schneider PD, Sugarbaker PH, Simpson C, Culnane M, Steinberg M. A prospective randomised trial of regional versus systemic continuous 5-fluoroxyuridine chemotherapy in the treatment of colorectal liver metastases. *Ann Surg* 1987;**206**:685-93.

26 Blair SD, Theodorou NA, Begent RHJ, Dawson PM, Salmon M, Riggs S, *et al*. Comparison of anti-foetal microvillus and anti-CEA antibodies in peroperative radioimmunolocalisation of colorectal cancer. *Br J Cancer* 1991;**61**:891-4.

Non-Hodgkin's lymphoma. I: Characterisation and treatment

SUSAN E O'REILLY, JOSEPH M CONNORS

The non-Hodgkin's lymphomas are a heterogeneous collection of lymphoproliferative malignancies whose clinical behaviour, prognosis, and management vary widely according to histological subtype, stage, and bulk of disease. They are the seventh most commonly diagnosed malignancy. Typically patients present with localised or generalised lymphadenopathy. Common presenting findings are haematological cytopenias, drenching night sweats, unexplained fevers, or weight loss greater than 10% of baseline (B symptoms); hepatosplenomegaly, abdominal masses, or compression of internal organs such as the gastrointestinal tract, blood vessels, airways, spinal cord, ureters, or bile ducts; or localised tumours of parenchymal or visceral organs. Nevertheless, lymphoma may mimic virtually any other neoplasm.

Until about 25 years ago, most patients with non-Hodgkin's lymphomas died of their disease. Although radiotherapy, single drug chemotherapy, and corticosteroid treatments were useful in palliating these patients, they were rarely curative. The advent of effective combination chemotherapy regimens, initially developed for Hodgkin's disease and subsequently applied to non-Hodgkin's lymphomas, resulted in the cure of advanced tumours in a few patients with lymphoma.[1] Similarly, improvements in histological subclassification, diagnostic radiology, radiation therapy, and general supportive care, especially in treating infectious complications of lymphomas, have all contributed to a better understanding of the nature of lymphomas and clearer planning of management of these disorders. More recently, developments in molecular biology of oncogenesis have begun to reveal the aetiological events in their development.[2]

Histological classification

Optimal management of non-Hodgkin's lymphomas must be based on a clear understanding of the cell pathology, the staging, and the clinical course of the various subtypes. A more detailed understanding of the prognostic factors influencing the course of lymphomas is also helpful in planning treatment. Several different histological classifications are used throughout the world, resulting in confusion and difficulty in comparing data from different centres. The working formulation for classifying lymphomas provides a comprehensive system which focuses on reproducing characteristics identifiable by light microscopy. It combines the most reproducible histological features in several classification schemes into a system allocating the lymphomas to 10 different subtypes, and it also provides a cross reference to other systems.[3] In the working formulation lymphomas are assigned to three categories—low, intermediate, and high grade—based on the natural course of these diseases, as modified by the best treatment available in the '60s and '70s.

The working formulation does not take into account the more detailed information now available on immunological phenotyping, which is based on specific cell membrane and cytoplasmic antigen testing and various DNA probe information. Such techniques are providing increasing insight into the molecular biological origin of lymphomas and have shown that the follicular (nodular) lymphomas are almost exclusively of B cell origin and that lymphoblastic lymphoma and mycosis fungoides typically arise from T cells. Diffuse lymphomas may arise from B or T cells or may be of indeterminate origin. We have used the working formulation terminology throughout this review (table I).

Developments in immunology, monoclonal antibody probes, cytogenetics, and characterisation of oncogenes and growth factors will continue to expand our understanding of lymphomas. And these added insights into lymphoma classification may eventually translate into improved treatments. Nevertheless, despite the increasing sophistication of the molecular biologists and pathologists most clinical decisions are based on light microscopy. An experienced haematopathologist can regularly and reproducibly distinguish between follicular (nodular) and diffuse lymph node disease and between small and large lymphocytes. It is usually relatively straightforward to distinguish the uncommon special lymphomas: small noncleaved cell (Burkitt's and non-Burkitt's) and T cell lymphoblastic lymphomas. In addition, haematopathologists can discriminate between the true lymphomas and lymphoma-like conditions such as sarcoidosis, syphilis, pseudolymphomas, and lymphadenopathy related to HIV, as well as rare conditions such as lymphomatoid granulomatosis, angioimmunoblastic lymphadenopathy, Wegener's granulomatosis, and lethal midline granuloma.

The prognostic and therapeutic implications of more recently defined entities such as intermediate cell lymphoma and its follicular variant, mantle zone lymphoma,[4] and peripheral T cell lymphoma (the commonest non-cutaneous T cell lymphoma)[5] are unclear at present and await more complete description and analysis. With current treatment techniques pathologists need only separate the lymphomas into three main therapeutic groups—low grade, aggressive (comprising the large cell lymphomas and immunoblastic lymphoma), and a special category (Burkitt's and non-Burkitt's small non cleaved cell lymphoma and T cell lymphoblastic lymphoma) to allow the clinician to plan treatment (table I). For planning treatment, immunoblastic lymphoma is best included in the same category as diffuse large cell lymphoma despite its assignment to the high grade group in the working formulation. The incidence, median age at diagnosis, distribution of stages, and natural course after treatment of different lymphomas are also summarised in table I.[3]

Staging

Staging has an important role in assigning prognosis and planning treatment in any patient with malignant lymphoma. Although the extent and duration of staging investigations may have to be modified in urgent situations or in frail patients, all other patients should undergo the mandatory procedures and any clinically indicated optional procedures listed in box 1. The most commonly used staging system is that of the Ann Arbor Conference (box 2).[6] This system was originally devised for Hodgkin's disease, a slowly progressive disease that tends to advance in an orderly fashion to contiguous, usually nodal structures. Malignant lymphomas, on the other hand, usually occur in elderly people, often progress early to distant nodal or extranodal sites, and may evolve rapidly. Therefore, the Ann Arbor

TABLE I — Correlation of the working formulation for classifying malignant lymphoma with treatment oriented approach. Clinical characteristics are derived from working formulation

Working formulation[1]	Treatment oriented approach	Relative frequency (%)	Median age at diagnosis (years)	Stage at diagnosis (%)		Male: female ratio	% With bone marrow disease	Median survival at 6 years	% Surviving 5 years
				I/II	III/IV				
Low grade	Low grade								
A — Small, lymphocytic		4	60	11	89	1·2	71	5·8	59
B — Follicular, small cleaved		23	54	18	82	1·3	51	7·2	70
C — Follicular, mixed large and small cleaved		8	56	27	73	0·8	30	5·1	50
Intermediate grade	Aggressive								
D — Follicular, large		4	55	27	73	1·8	34	3·0	45
E — Diffuse, small cleaved		7	58	28	72	1	32	3·4	33
F — Diffuse, mixed large and small cleaved		7	58	45	55	1·1	14	2·7	38
G — Diffuse, large		20	57	46	54	1	10	2·7	38
High grade	Special								
H — Immunoblastic		8	51	52	48	1·5	12	1·3	32
I — Lymphoblastic		4	17	27	73	2	50	2·0	26
J — Small, non-cleaved		5	30	34	66	2·6	14	0·7	23

Box 1 — Staging procedures for malignant lymphomas

Mandatory procedures

History and physical examination
Biopsy of diagnostic tissue
Laboratory profile:
  Complete blood count, liver and renal function tests, serum calcium concentration, serum protein electrophoresis
Chest radiographs
Computed tomography of abdomen and pelvis
Bone marrow aspiration and biopsy
Upper gastrointestinal series, small bowel follow through for all ear, nose, and throat lymphomas (in 20% of such lymphomas there is gastrointestinal disease)
Ear, nose, and throat examination (to visualise Waldeyer's ring, nasopharynx) in all gastrointestinal lymphomas

Optional procedures

Lymphangiography (only if result will alter treatment)
Cytology of cerebrospinal fluid in high risk patients:
  Small non-cleaved and lymphoblastic tumours
  Large cell tumour with marrow or sinus disease
  Patients with neurological abnormalities
Cytology of pleural or peritoneal effusions
Computed tomography or radiography of symptomatic sites
Bone scanning (if pain present)
Laparotomy recommended for:
  Diagnosis of abdominal mass
  Resection of gastrointestinal lymphoma

---

staging system is not as useful a predictor of treatment outcome in malignant lymphoma as in Hodgkin's disease. As a consequence, a simple staging system based on anatomic extent of disease, tumour bulk, and constitutional symptoms is adequate for initial clinical decision making. This system is based on the Ann Arbor staging system plus information about the patient's age and bulk of disease (box 3) and applies to a wide range of presentations of lymphoma.

Once a pathologist has reviewed a biopsy specimen from a lymph node or extranodal site affected by lymphoma and clinical staging has been completed as described above, patients can be classified for treatment according to histology, extent of disease, and age. Table II gives guidelines for an overall approach to management.

Box 2—Ann Arbor staging classification for Hodgkin's disease

Stage I
Single lymph node region affected or single extralymphatic organ or site

Stage II
Two or more lymph node regions affected on the same side of the diaphragm with or without localised disease in extralymphatic site (IIE)

Stage III
Lymph node regions affected on both sides of the diaphragm with or without localised disease of an extralymphatic organ or site (IIIE) or spleen (IIIS), or both (IIISE)

Stage IV
Diffuse or disseminated disease in one or more extralymphatic organs, with or without associated lymph node disease

Subtype A—Asymptomatic

Subtype B—Patient has constitutional symptoms:
  Fever, night sweats, or weight loss >10% of baseline

Low grade lymphomas

About 40% of lymphomas encountered in North America and western Europe are low grade. Box 4 shows their characteristics. These lymphomas typically present insidiously, often with progressive lymphadenopathy, which may wax and wane, or with cytopenias,

---

Box 3—Simplified staging system for clinical decision making

Limited stage	*Advanced stage*
Ann Arbor stage I or II	Ann Arbor stage III or IV
and	or
Absence of B symptoms	Presence of B symptoms
and	or
Largest tumour diameter <10 cm	Mass >10 cm

TABLE II—Guidelines for treatment of malignant lymphoma

Category	Histology	Stage	Age (years)	Treatment
Low grade	Small, lymphocytic Follicular, small cleaved	Limited	All	Radiation of affected site
	Follcular, mixed	Advanced	All	Observation if asymptomatic and without threatening disease Single drug chemotherapy if gradual response sufficient Multi-drug chemotherapy if rapid response necessary Local irradiation for focally troublesome disease Enrolment on aggressive experimental protocols
Aggressive	Diffuse, small cleaved Diffuse, mixed	Limited	All	Brief chemotherapy and irradiation of affected site
	Follicular, large Diffuse, large Immunoblastic	Advanced	<70	Frequency of dose intensive chemotherapy
			≥70	Chemotherapy modified to maximum tolerable toxicity
Special	Lymphoblastic Small nonocleaved	All	<60	High dose intensive chemotherapy with central nervous system chemoprophylaxis
			≥60	Palliative chemotherapy and irradiation

hepatosplenomegaly, or compression of ureters, veins, or bile ducts. Patients usually do not have typical B symptoms. Careful staging is worth while to identify the minority of patients who have limited stage disease in whom radiation of the affected site may be curative. Up to 50% of patients with limited stage disease (I or IIA, low bulk) will achieve long term freedom from disease, although whether they have been cured or will have late relapses remains to be established.[7] In most patients with low grade lymphoma who have advanced stage disease, management is determined by the severity of symptoms and the degree to which organs are compromised. Traditionally, asymptomatic patients with normal blood counts, no actual or imminent organ compromise, and no cosmetically unacceptable masses may be observed safely until symptomatic or threatening disease develops. Local problems can often be dealt with by irradiation. Systemic problems merit chemotherapy, the choice of which depends on the urgency with which a response must be achieved.

Non-urgent response

If it is not necessary to obtain a rapid response, oral chlorambucil or

---

Box 4—Clinical characteristics of lymphomas

Low grade	*Aggressive histology*
Patients' median age 55 to 60 years (rarely <40)	Patients' median age 55 years
Indolent disease with median survival ≥7 years	Firm, fixed lymph nodes
Limited stage (10%)—potentially curable	Potentially curable
Advanced stage (90%)—currently incurable	Invasion of adjacent tissues
Do not usually invade adjacent soft tissue	Often affects unusual extranodal structures, including central nervous system, lung, soft tissue, bone, testes, and gastrointestinal tract
Do not usually invade central nervous system, testes	Early systemic metastases, even when apparently localised
Bone marrow disease in 50% of cases	

---

cyclophosphamide with or without prednisone is the best treatment. The main side effect with this approach is cumulative marrow suppression, especially if treatment is given daily, but treatment is usually well tolerated. Prednisone can be a useful treatment initially, but prolonged use is best avoided because of its side effects, which can be cumulative and troublesome, particularly in elderly patients.

When oral chemotherapy is used the white blood cell count must be monitored regularly. If it remains in the normal range the dose of the drug should be increased to ensure that a sufficient amount is being absorbed. Oral therapy should not be deemed ineffective until the dose delivered is capable of causing mild myelosuppression.

Prednisone should be used alone for treating patients with severe anaemia, myelosuppression, or thrombocytopenia due to a packed marrow or immune destruction. A reasonable dose is 40 mg/m^2 daily. An alkylating drug such as chlorambucil or cyclophosphamide can be cautiously introduced after an initial response and prednisone gradually reduced.

Cytopenias related to immune destruction may be encountered in diffuse small lymphocytic lymphoma (which has a clinical course similar to that of chronic lymphatic leukaemia), or occasionally other diffuse lymphomas, but are rarely seen in the follicular lymphomas.

Urgent response

If a rapid response is needed in an advanced low grade lymphoma then combination chemotherapy is indicated. Since these lymphomas are very responsive to alkylating agents, combinations including cyclophosphamide, vincristine, and prednisone with or without additional drugs are popular and reasonable (table II). Patients should be treated until a sustained complete response or stabilisation is achieved.

Radiotherapy is a useful adjunct to the palliative treatment of low grade lymphomas. The extent of disease should dictate whether radiotherapy is of only the affected site or of an extended field. The decision to use wide field radiotherapy must be balanced against the potential for the associated myelosuppression to compromise later delivery of systemic chemotherapy.

Experimental treatment of advanced stage low grade lymphoma

Low grade lymphoma is a chronic disease which in the past had a median survival of eight to 10 years but inevitably proved fatal. It remains difficult to manage, especially in younger patients. Several experimental programmes are evaluating the benefit of aggressive treatment after diagnosis in younger patients.[8-11] Some centres offer newly diagnosed patients autologous or allogeneic bone marrow transplantation immediately after diagnosis. At the British Columbia Cancer Agency newly diagnosed patients with advanced stage disease are offered an experimental protocol comprising 12 weeks of intensive outpatient chemotherapy followed by radiotherapy to all originally affected lymph nodes.[12] The National Cancer Institute treats such patients with multidrug chemotherapy and radiotherapy.[11] All of these studies show an initial improvement in disease free survival and freedom from further treatment for low grade lymphoma, but longer follow up will be needed to establish whether patients are cured of their disease or whether disease free survival or overall survival is improved by early aggressive intervention. Until these experimental programmes have longer term results the conventional management of low grade lymphomas described earlier in this chapter remains the standard.

Limited stage large cell lymphoma

As defined previously, limited stage disease includes Ann Arbor stage I or II disease, a tumour mass <10 cm, and the absence of B symptoms. Historically, these patients were treated with only radiotherapy; however, the reported cure rate with such local treatment varied between 25% and 75% but averaged less than 50%.[13-15]

Since combination chemotherapy cures advanced disease it seemed reasonable to use the initial management of early stage disease.[16-20] The advantage of this approach is that the chemotherapy can be quite brief, lessening the disruption of the patient's life and minimising cumulative side effects. Most importantly, the chemotherapy is given when it is most likely to be effective, rather than late in the disease course when the tumour has had time to evolve clones of drug resistant cells.

The current recommendations for limited stage disease are that patients receive combination chemotherapy with or without irradiation of the affected site. During 1980-4 Connors et al treated 78 patients with three cycles of chemotherapy with cyclophosphamide, doxorubicin, vincristine, and prednisone (CHOP) plus irradiation of affected sites.[21] This well tolerated regimen cured more than 80% of these patients. The approach has been refined to six weeks of weekly chemotherapy with doxorubicin, cyclophosphamide, vincristine, bleomycin, and prednisone (ACOB), with similar results.[22] The excellent outcome with such brief chemotherapy means that it is the optimal treatment irrespective of age in patients with early stage disease. It is uncertain whether radiotherapy adds to the overall outcome, as no trials have yet been published.

Advanced stage, aggressive histology (large cell) lymphomas

Lymphomas with aggressive histology (follicular large, diffuse cleaved, non-cleaved, diffuse mixed, and immunoblastic lymphomas) comprise about 40% of all lymphomas (box 4). This group of large cell lymphomas is highly responsive to combination chemotherapy and a proportion of all patients may be cured with this treatment. Early regimens developed for treating Hodgkin's disease, such as mustine, vincristine, procarbazine, and prednisone (MOPP), resulted in the first reported cures of advanced stage diffuse large cell lymphoma.[1 23 24] Subsequently, the addition of doxorubicin proved highly effective in obtaining complete responses in these lymphomas. Studies of the CHOP regimen have reported a 30% overall 10 year survival in advanced stage disease.[25 26] Other first generation combinations have produced similar results. Many different regimens have

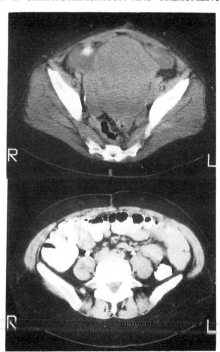

Figure 1–Computed tomograms showing (above) enormous large cell lymphoma filling the pelvis and obliterating bowel loops and bladder and (below) dramatic resolution of the tumour six weeks later after initiation of chemotherapy with MACOP-B

since been developed which give more intensive treatment and additional drugs. Toxicity is increased, particularly from infection, but it remains unclear whether the efficacy of treatment is improved. Several regimens, such as m-BACOD, ProMACE-Cytabom, and MACOP-B (figures 1 and 2), have been reported to improve survival in single institution studies,[27-30] and randomised clinical trials to evaluate the relative effectiveness of these different regimens are ongoing or recently completed. The results of well designed large randomised studies will be important in determining management of aggressive histology lymphomas in the 1990s. For the present, in view of the persisting controversy over which is the best treatment approach, we recommend that clinicians select the regimen with which they feel most comfortable and in which they have the most confidence and that it is used in maximally tolerated doses.

Prognostic factors in diffuse large cell lymphoma

Several studies of prognostic factors for outcome have been

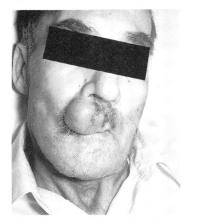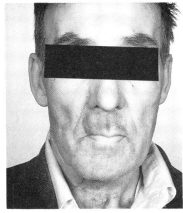

Figure 2—(Left) Patient with a diffuse large cell lymphoma of the upper lip and soft tissues of the cheek and (right) three weeks later after multi-agent chemotherapy

published. In particular, data from Coiffier et al,[31] Shipp et al,[32] Jagannath et al,[33] and Hoskins et al,[34] have pointed to a constellation of factors which predict an adverse prognosis. In aggregate these factors include age over 60, a poor performance status, a lactate dehydrogenase concentration greater than three times normal, tumour bulk >10 cm, the presence of B symptoms, disease of two or more extranodal sites, multiple nodal sites affected, and various other less common factors such as a low serum albumin concentration. Various formulas to predict which patients will fail are now being developed and more intensive treatments with either bone marrow transplantation protocols or intensive chemotherapy with cytokine support will probably be designed to treat patients young enough to withstand more aggressive treatment who have a predictably poor outcome with current standard chemotherapy regimens. One of the challenges facing lymphoma specialists in the next 10 years is to define the precise subgroups of patients in whom such treatment is indicated and then to develop modifications of current treatment programmes and prove whether they result in a better outcome.

1 Lowenbraun S, DeVita VT, Serpick AA. Combination chemotherapy with nitrogen mustard, vincristine, procarbazine, and prednisone in lymphosarcoma and reticulum cell sarcoma. Cancer 1970;25:1018.
2 Weinberg RA. Oncogenes and the mechanisms of carcinogenesis. Sci Am 1987;12(2):1.
3 National Cancer Institute. Sponsored study of classification of non-Hodgkin's lymphomas. Summary and description of a working formulation for clinical usage. Cancer 1982;49:2112.

4 Weisenburger DD, Kim H, Rappaport H. Mantle zone lymphoma: a follicular variant of intermediate lymphoma. *Cancer* 1982;**49**:2112.

5 Greer JP, York JC, Cousar JB Mitchel RT, Flexner JM, Collins RD, *et al.* Peripheral T cell lymphoma: a clinicopathologic study of 42 cases. *J Clin Oncol* 1984;**2**:7.

6 Carbone PP, Kaplan HS, Musshoff K, Smithers DW, Tubiana M. Report of the committee on Hodgkin's disease staging classification. *Cancer Res* 1971;**31**:1860.

7 Gospodarowicz MK, Bush RS, Brown TC, Chua TC. Prognostic factors in nodular lymphomas: a multivariate analysis based on the Princess Margaret Hospital experience. *Int J Rad Oncol Biol Phys* 1984;**10**(4):489.

8 Glick JH, Barnes JM, Ezdinli EZ, Berard CW, Orlon EL, Bennett JM. Nodular mixed lymphoma: results of a randomized trial failing to confirm prolonged disease-free survival with COPP chemotherapy. *Blood* 1981;**58**: 920.

9 Longo DL, Young RC, Hubbard SM, Wesley M, Fisher RL, Jaffe E, *et al.* Prolonged initial remission in patients with nodular mixed lymphoma. *Ann Intern Med* 1984;**100**:651.

10 McLaughlin P, Fuller LM, Velasquez WS, Butler JJ, Hagemeister FB, Sullivan-Holley JA, *et al.* Stage III follicular lymphoma: durable remissions with a combined chemotherapy-radiotherapy regimen. *J Clin Oncol* 1987;**5**: 867.

11 Young RC, Longo DL, Glatstein E, Matis LA, Ostchega Y, Nanfro J, *et al.* Watchful-waiting (WW) *v* aggressive combined modality therapy (Rx) in the treatment of Stage III-IV indolent non-Hodgkin's lymphoma [abstract]. *Proceedings of the American Society of Clinical Oncology* 1987;**6**:A790.

12 Klasa RJ, Hoskins PJ, O'Reilly SE, Fairey R, Voss N, Gascoyne R. *et al.* BP-VACOP and extensive lymph node irradiation (RT) for advanced stage low grade lymphoma. *Proceedings of the American Society of Clinical Oncology* 1992;**11**:328.

13 Jones SE, Fuks Z, Kaplan HS, Rosenberg SA. Non-Hodgkin's lymphomas. V. Rsults of radiotherapy. *Cancer* 1973;**32**:682.

14 Vokes EE, Ultmann JE, Golomb HM, Gaynor ER, Ferguson DJ, Griem ML, *et al.* Lonterm survival of patients with localized diffuse histiocytic lymphoma. *J Clin Oncol* 1985;**3**:1309.

15 Levitt SH, Lee CKK, Bloomfield CD, Frizzera G. The role of radiation therapy in the treatment of early stage large cell lymphoma. *Hematol Oncol* 1985;**3**:33.

16 Nissen NI, Ersboll J, Hansen HS, Walbom-Jorgensen S, Pederson-Bjergaard J, Hansen HM, *et al.* A randomized study of radiotherapy versus radiotherapy plus chemotherapy in stage I-II non-Hodgkin's lymphomas. *Cancer* 1983; **52**:1.

17 Landberg TG, Hakansson LG, Moller TR, Mattisson WKI, Landys KE, Johansson BG, *et al.* CVP remission maintenance in stage I or II non-Hodgkin's lymphomas: preliminary results of a randomised study. *Cancer* 1979;**44**:831.

18 Monfardini S, Banfi A, Bonadonna G, Rilke F, Milani F, Valagussa P, *et al.* Improved five year survival after combined radiotherapy-chemotherapy for stage I-II non-Hodgkin's lymphomas. *Int J Radiat Oncol Biol Phys* 1980;**6**:125.

19 Miller TP, Jones SE. Initial chemotherapy for clinically staged localized non-Hodgkin's lymphomas of unfavorable histology. In: Ford RJ, Fuller LM, Hagenmeister FB, eds. *Hodgkin's disease and non-Hodgkin's lymphoma: new perspectives in immunopathology, diagnosis and treatment.* New York: Raven Press, 1984:33-9.

20 Cabanillas F. Chemotherapy as definitive treatment of stage I-II large cell and diffuse mixed lymphomas. *Hematol Oncol* 1985;**3**:25.

21 Connors JM, Klimo P, Fairey RN, Voss N. Brief chemotherapy and involved field radiation therapy for limited stage aggressive histology lymphoma. *Ann Intern Med* 1987;**107**:25.

22 Connors JM, Fairey R, Klimo P, O'Reilly S, Voss N. ACOB: 6-week chemotherapy and involved field radiotherapy (IFRT) for limited stage large cell lymphoma, initial results. *Proceedings of the American Society of Clinical Oncology.* 1988;**7**:224.

23 Luce JK, Gamble JF, Wilson HE, Monto RN, Isaacs BL, Palmer RL, *et al.* Combined cyclophosphamide, vincristine and prednisone therapy of malignant lymphoma. *Cancer* 1971;**28**:306.

24 Bagley CM, DeVita VT Jr, Berard CW, Canellos GP. Advanced lymphosarcoma: intensive cyclical combination chemotherapy with cyclophosphamide, vincristine and prednisone. *Ann Intern Med* 1972;**76**:227.

25 Armitage JO, Fyfe MAE, Lewis J. Long-term remission durability and functional status of patients treated for diffuse histiocytic lymphoma with the CHOP regimens. *J Clin Oncol* 1984;**2**:898.

26 Coltman CA Jr, Dahlberg S, Jones SE. CHOP is curative in thirty percent of patients with large

cell lymphoma: a twelve year Southwest Oncology Group follow up. In: Skarin AT, ed. *Update on treatment for diffuse large cell lymphoma*. New York: John Wiley, 1986:71-7.

27 Skarin AT, Canellos GP, Rosenthal DS, Case DC, MacIntyre JM, Pinkus GS, *et al.* Improved prognosis of diffuse histiocytic and undifferentiated lymphoma by use of high dose methotrexate alternating with standard agents (M-BACOD). *J Clin Oncol* 1983;**1**:91.

28 Skarin AT, Canellos GP, Rosenthal DS, Case D, McIntyre J, Pinkus C, *et al.* Moderate dose methotrexate (m) combined with bleomycin (B), Adriamycin (A), cyclophosphamide (C), Oncovin (O), and dexamethasone (D), m-BACOD is advanced diffuse histiocytic lymphoma (DHL) [abstract]. *Proceedings of the American Society of Clinical Oncology* 1983;**2**:220.

29 Longo DL, DeVita VT, Duffey PL, Wesley MN, Ihde DC, Hubbard SM, *et al.* Superiority of ProMACE-CytaBOM over ProMACE-MOPP in the treatment of advanced diffuse aggressive lymphoma: results of a prospective randomized trial. *J Clin Oncol* 1991;**9**:25.

30 Klimo P, Connors JM. MACOP-B chemotherapy for the treatment of diffuse large cell lymphoma. *Ann Intern Med* 1985;**102**:596.

31 Coiffier B, LePage E. Prognosis of aggressive lymphomas: a study of five prognostic models with patients included in the LNH-84 regimen. *Blood* 1989;**74**:558.

32 Shipp MA, Harrington DP, Klatt MK, Jochelson MS, Pinkus GS, Marshall JL, *et al.* Identification of major prognostic subgroups of patients with large cell lymphoma treated with m-BACOD or M-BACOD. *Ann Intern Med* 1986;**104**:757.

33 Jagannath S, Velasquez WS, Tucker SL, Fuller LM, McLaughlin PW, Manning JT, *et al.* Tumor burden assessment and its implication for a prognostic model in advanced diffuse large cell lymphoma. *J Clin Oncol* 1986;**4**:859.

34 Hoskins PJ, Ng V, Spinelli J, Klimo P, Connors JM. Prognostic variables in patients with diffuse large-cell lymphoma treated with MACOP-B. *J Clin Oncol* 1991;**9**:220.

Non-Hodgkin's lymphoma. II: Management problems

SUSAN E O'REILLY, JOSEPH M CONNORS

In the previous chapter we discussed identification, staging, and basic management.[1] In this chapter we discuss some of the conditions which present management problems and appropriate treatment of special and rare lymphomas.

Problems in treating aggressive lymphomas

Elderly patients

Lymphomas are primarily diseases of older patients; 60% of all patients are aged 60 or more. Some newly diagnosed patients are either too old or too frail to undergo the aggressive treatment regimens used in younger patients. Older patients experience greater toxicity, a worse outcome, and are underrepresented in reported clinical trials in diffuse large cell lymphoma.

In general, older patients should be treated with curative intent unless they have a serious intercurrent illness that precludes combination chemotherapy. Treatment must be tailored to fit their age and stage of disease. Patients with limited stage disease will usually tolerate the standard brief chemotherapy with or without radiotherapy which is appropriate for all patients and all ages.[1]

Patients presenting with advanced stage disease may be treated either with CHOP (cyclophosphamide, vincristine, procarbazine, and prednisone) protocols in which doses are modified initially and then adjusted according to toxicity as described by the Nebraska Lymphoma Group[2] or with protocols developed specifically for older patients. We have reported on two regimens specifically designed for patients aged over 65, low dose ACOP-B (cyclophosphamide, doxorubicin, vincristine, prednisone, and bleomycin) and VABE (vincristine, doxorubicin, bleomycin, etoposide, prednisone),[3] and more recently have evolved an even briefer five treatment, eight week regimen called POCE.[4] The results with this treatment programme are similar to those seen with the two previous regimens and the treatment is briefer. Five year survival of 133 patients treated with any one of these three regimens designed for older patients was 38%, which compares favourably with the 44% survival achieved in patients aged 60 to 70 years treated with our centre's aggressive protocols for younger patients. Giving more aggressive treatment to older patients has not been shown to yield a significant improvement in survival and can cause excessive toxicity. As patients aged 60-70 do not seem to have a much better outcome with more aggressive treatment we are reassured that our specially designed programmes are not undertreating older patients.

Follicular large and diffuse small cleaved cell lymphoma

These uncommon lymphomas are usually grouped with the aggressive histology lymphomas and often are also managed in the same way. Unfortunately, their clinical behaviour is not as consistent as that of other large cell lymphomas and the outcome is often similar to that in low grade disease, in which patients follow a chronic relapsing pattern. Management of these diseases is best designed for the individual and the patient should be treated according to the pre-existing clinical course. In younger patients treatment as for aggressive histology lymphoma is reasonable, but in older patients, in whom the disease often follows an indolent course, expectant management or alkylating drugs are appropriate.

Discordant, transformed, and composite lymphomas

In patients with discordant lymphomas, both aggressive histology disease and low grade disease are detected in separate areas—for example, small cleaved cell lymphoma in the bone marrow and simultaneous large cell lymphoma in a peripheral lymph node. Transformed lymphoma is an aggressive lymphoma developing in a patient with a pre-existing history of low grade lymphoma. Composite lymphoma is the coexistence of an aggressive lymphoma and a low grade lymphoma in the same site (usually a lymph node). These three examples of two separate types of lymphomas coexisting in the same patient should not be confused with the mixed large and small cell lymphomas in which a single histological subtype contains two different sized malignant cells. The guiding principle in managing discordant, composite, and transformed lymphomas is to try to eradicate the most aggressive component of this disease since this constitutes the greatest threat to survival. Thus, treatment is usually the same as described for large cell lymphoma.[1]

Newly diagnosed patients with discordant or composite lymphomas generally have a favourable short term prognosis, similar to that for patients with only large cell disease. Nevertheless, if patients survive the aggressive component of their disease they remain at risk of having the indolent component slowly re-emerge. The prognosis in patients with a transformed lymphoma depends both on the usual prognostic factors (age, stage, performance status, bulk of disease, etc) and on the extent and toxicity of earlier treatment for the low grade disease. Patients who have been heavily pretreated or have low grade disease that is refractory to chemotherapy are unlikely to tolerate or respond to aggressive treatment. In these circumstances treatment should be tailored to the individual and given with palliative intent.

Special sites of lymphoma

Gastrointestinal lymphoma

Gastrointestinal lymphomas may be complicated by a haemorrhage or perforation of a stomach or intestinal tumour in up to 25% of patients.[4 5] In addition, the rapid liquefaction of a treated lymphoma may expose blood vessels or result in a full thickness perforation of the bowel wall. Either of these life threatening problems may occur at any time during treatment and require surgical intervention.

If a patient has a localised resectable gastrointestinal tumour a laparotomy and complete resection should be attempted. This facilitates diagnosis and debulking and avoids the complications of haemorrhage or perforation. Surgery is contraindicated if the patient is too frail or if complete resection of the tumour is either technically impossible or would be so extensive as to compromise the patient's nutrition or unduly delay systemic treatment. As a rule total gastrectomy or major small bowel resection that would result in the short bowel syndrome should be avoided. Patients who are malnourished because of gastrointestinal lymphoma may require intravenous hyperalimentation while being treated.

After resection, or if resection is not feasible, patients should be treated as described for either advanced stage or limited stage disease.[1] Chemotherapy is mandatory for all such patients who have large cell lymphoma. All patients with local gastrointestinal lymphoma should have a detailed ear, nose, and throat examination to rule out occult disease. There is about a 20% risk of Waldeyer's ring also being affected, and this may indicate the need for extensive treatment.

Head and neck disease

All patients with affected tonsils, adenoids, pharynx, or tongue should have a complete contrast study of the stomach and intestine to detect gastrointestinal disease (figs 1 and 2). About 20% of patients presenting with primary disease of Waldeyer's ring will have occult gastrointestinal disease.

If paranasal or basilar skull sinuses are affected there is an increased risk that the central nervous system will be affected.[5] This risk may be as high as 50% and necessitates prophylaxis. In patients with localised large cell lymphoma of the sinuses one practical approach is to give treatment in three phases: brief chemotherapy, followed by radiation of the affected site, and finally intrathecal chemotherapy.

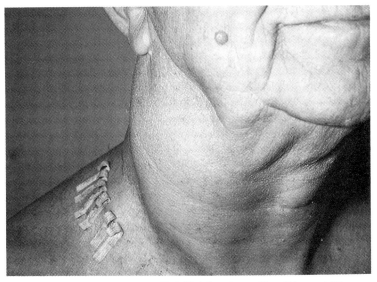

Figure 1—Neck of patient with non-Hodgkin's lymphoma. Site of biopsy visible

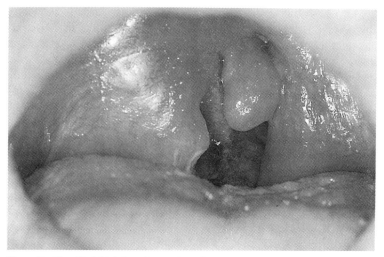

Figure 2—Non-Hodgkin's lymphoma of tonsils

Testicular lymphomas

The incidence of testicular lymphoma increases with age, becoming the most common testicular malignancy in men over 60. In general, lymphomas at this site are treated according to stage except that the scrotum should always be irradiated as there is a high risk of bilaterality and the testis may act as a sanctuary from cytotoxic drugs.

Central nervous system lymphoma

Lymphoma may affect the leptomeninges or parenchyma of the brain, in isolation or as part of systemic disease. Leptomeningeal metastases occur with variable frequency depending on the other sites of disease; the risk is highest with paranasal sinuses (50%) and bone marrow disease (10-20%) in patients with intermediate or high grade lymphoma. Leptomeningeal disease is extremely rare in patients with low grade lymphoma.

Patients with established leptomeningeal disease have a poor prognosis but occasionally can be cured. An Ommaya reservoir connected by a catheter to a lateral ventricle facilitates the giving of intrathecal chemotherapy with methotrexate or cytosine arabinoside, or both. We usually give chemotherapy until at least six treatments beyond a complete cytological remission in the cerebrospinal fluid.

As patients with affected paranasal sinuses, peripheral blood, or bone marrow are at increased risk of spread to the meninges they should receive prophylactic intrathecal chemotherapy. One approach is to give six doses, two each week, after the systemic disease has completely responded to treatment. This approach often has cumulative toxicity with concurrent systemic chemotherapy and must be given with care.

Primary lymphoma of the brain is rare (1% of all lymphomas). In most cases the histology is aggressive —usually large cell or small non-cleaved cell. This presentation of lymphoma is commonly seen in association with HIV infection or organ immunosuppression after transplantation and in these cases is probably related to Epstein-Barr virus. Presentation is often insidious and this disease may easily be misdiagnosed in elderly patients. Systemic disease is rare when the initial presentation is a mass lesion in the brain.

The prognosis is poor despite an initial response to corticosteroids and radiotherapy and most patients succumb within one year of diagnosis, either from recurrent tumour or from neurological complications of the disease and its treatment. Overall, the two year disease free survival is less than 20%, and it is unclear whether systemic chemotherapy improves the prognosis for patients with primary brain lymphoma. The outcome for patients with AIDS remains even poorer and treatment is often palliative.

Lymphoma associated with aids

Patients with AIDS have an increased risk of developing aggressive lymphomas (usually large cell, immunoblastic, or small non-cleaved cell types). It is reasonable to screen patients presenting with these subtypes of lymphoma for HIV infection. Knowledge of infection is useful in planning treatment, estimating prognosis, and managing infectious complications. In addition, knowledge of the prevalence of AIDS in the population of patients treated for lymphoma is essential in interpreting the results of clinical trials since these patients generally have a worse outcome and experience more toxicity.

Although a few patients with AIDS related lymphomas may achieve a sustained complete remission, unfortunately, almost all patients eventually die of either the malignancy or AIDS related complications. At present the median survival of such patients is less than six months. Nevertheless, patients with AIDS who do not have a history of previous severe opportunistic infection and whose performance status is good may respond well to chemotherapy and achieve durable remissions. Optimal treatment should be delivered as long as tolerance is adequate. In general, however, treatment of AIDS related lymphomas remains palliative because of the poor prognosis of the underlying infectious disease.

Recurrent large cell lymphoma

Even the most effective treatment regimens for large cell lymphoma cure only about 50-60% of patients with advanced stage disease. Patients who are refractory to treatment or relapse after treatment often require further chemotherapy or radiotherapy. Several salvage regimens such as IMVP-16 (ifosfamide, methotrexate, etoposide),[7] MIME (methyl gag, ifosfamide, methotrexate, etoposide)[8] and DHAP (cisplatin, cytosine arabinoside, dexamethasone)[9] have been developed and produced some long term survivors. However, patients often relapse again and only a few achieve durable remission. Similarly, bone marrow transplantation protocols developed for relapsing diffuse large cell lymphoma induce high response rates, but less than 20% of patients achieve durable disease free survival.[10] Only a few patients even proceed to such aggressive treatments and the overall outcome for relapsing patients with diffuse large cell lymphoma remains very poor.

Clearly, further research is needed on the initial management of patients identified as having poor prognostic factors if a higher cure rate is to be achieved in the initial treatment of aggressive lymphoma.

Special lymphomas

Special lymphomas are uncommon, rapidly proliferative diseases which constitute less than 10% of all lymphomas. They require intensive treatments similar to that used for acute leukaemia, including prophylactic treatment of the central nervous system.

Lymphoblastic lymphoma

Lymphoblastic lymphoma is a disease usually seen in children or young adults (median age 17 years). It is twice as common in males as females, onset is usually rapid, a mediastinal mass is common, and B symptoms and bone marrow or central nervous diseases are often found. Malignant cells are usually, but not invariably, phenotypically T cell.

Coleman et al have developed a predictive model based on the results with multiagent chemotherapy (cyclophosphamide, doxorubicin, vincristine, prednisone, L-asparaginase, central nervous system prophylaxis, methotrexate, and mercaptopurine).[11] This identifies patients with a good prognosis (bone marrow not affected, normal lactate dehydrogenase concentration), who have an 80% cure rate, and a second group with a poor prognosis, in which only 20% are cured. In our experience the overall outcome for all young patients presenting with this diagnosis is not as good as that reported by Coleman *et al*. Very aggressive initial treatment including upfront autologous or allogeneic bone marrow transplantation is valid for this disease. Further experimental treatments need to be tested in these patients to establish standard management.

Small non-cleaved cell lymphoma

Small non-cleaved cell lymphoma is also labelled as diffuse undifferentiated lymphoma in the Rappaport classification. It is a B cell neoplasm which is highly mitotic and rapidly proliferative. The age distribution is biphasic; the Burkitt type is seen more often in younger patients and the non-Burkitt type more often in older patients. Abdominal or gastrointestinal presentations are typical. These diseases are potentially curable when found in early stages but are difficult to eradicate in more advanced stages in the adult population. Although these lymphomas usually respond to high dose chemotherapy with alkylating drugs such as cyclophosphamide, rapid expression of drug resistance, relapse, and death often result.

Regimens similar to that reported by the United States National Cancer Institute are usually used for treating small non-cleaved cell lymphomas of both varieties.[12] No satisfactory treatment for the majority of patients with bulky disease has been identified. Such patients should be referred to institutions where new approaches are being investigated. Again high dose chemoradiotherapy and bone marrow transplantation in first remission should be considered in younger patients.

Although lymphoblastic lymphoma and small non-cleaved cell lymphoma arise from different lymphocyte cell lines (T and B respectively) and although there are important variations in the regimens used to treat them, they have some important features in common. Patients are at high risk of the acute tumour lysis syndrome when initially treated, especially those who have bulky disease or already impaired renal function. This may cause death from cardiac arrest secondary to the metabolic consequences of hyperuricaemia, renal failure, hyperkalaemia, hyperphosphataemia, and hypocal aemia. All patients should be pretreated with allopurinol and sodium bicarbonate, a high fluid output should be established before treatment, and preparation should be made for haemodialysis in patients thought to be at risk of renal failure (particularly patients with a raised lactate dehydrogenase concentration). Central nervous system and bone marrow disease are common in both lymphomas and central nervous system prophylaxis is indicated. Small non-cleaved cell lymphoma is the most common lymphoma seen in immunosuppressed patients such as those with AIDS, organ transplants, or congenital immunodeficiency. Treatment of such patients is complicated by the underlying immunodeficiency and is seldom successful without correction of that defect. Recipients of organ transplants may also develop lymphoma-like lymphoproliferations which may resolve on withdrawal of immunosuppressants.[13]

Miscellaneous lymphomas and related conditions

The following lymphoproliferative malignancies are reviewed briefly in order to place them in context relative to the malignant lymphomas.

B cell neoplasms

Chronic lymphatic leukaemia is an indolent disease, typically occurring in elderly people and associated with long survival. It is morphologically indistinguishable from small lymphocytic lymphoma and is managed in the same way.

Waldenström's macroglobulinaemia is the plasmacytoid variant of small lymphocytic lymphoma and is associated with an IgM paraprotein. Management is as for small lymphocytic lymphoma. Patients with this variant may develop symptomatic hyperviscosity. This is usually best managed with plasmapheresis and institution of chemotherapy with an alkylating drug such as cyclophosphamide or chlorambucil.

Multiple myeloma is a malignancy of mature plasma cells which primarily affects bones and bone marrow and is usually associated with a monoclonal gammopathy in the blood or urine. The clinical course is often complicated by bacterial infections, renal disease, hypercalcaemia, pancytopenia, and localised bone destruction. This disease is usually treated with oral alkylating drugs and prednisone with irradiation of focally symptomatic bone lesions.

Intermediate cell lymphocytic lymphoma has cytological features between those of small lymphocytic (well differentiated) and small

Management problems in patients with non-Hodgkin's lymphoma

- Elderly patients with aggressive lymphomas experience greater toxicity and a worse outcome from treatment

- Gastrointestinal lymphomas may be complicated by haemorrhage or perforation

- In testicular lymphoma the scrotum should always be irradiated because of a high risk of bilateral disease and the possibility of the testis acting as a sanctuary from cytotoxic drugs

- Even the most effective regimens for large cell lymphomas cure only about a half of patients with advanced disease

- The acute tumour lysis syndrome, which follows initial treatment particularly of bulky tumours, may result in death from the metabolic consequences of hyperuricaemia, renal failure, hyperkalaemia, hyperphosphataemia, and hypocalcaemia

cleaved cell (poorly differentiated) lymphoma and includes so called "mantle zone" lymphoma.[13] Typically, patients present with advanced disease and may have a shorter survival than patients with low grade lymphoma. The nodal architecture is usually, but not invariably, diffuse. These patients are best managed in the same manner as those with diffuse small cleaved cell lymphoma. Mantle zone lymphomas are intermediate cell lymphomas in which the malignant cells proliferate in wide mantles around germinal centres that appear normal. They are a follicular variant of intermediate lymphocytic lymphoma and usually are more aggressive than small cleaved cell lymphomas. In the working formulation intermediate cell and mantle zone lymphomas are usually included in the small cleaved cell or mixed cell categories and are not separately described. A better definition and more reproducible identification of these uncommon lymphomas will improve our understanding of their natural course.

T cell neoplasms

Mycosis fungoides and its variant, the Sézary syndrome, are rare cutaneous T cell lymphomas which may resemble eczema or psoriasis in early presentation. These diseases usually progress gradually to formation of plaques and tumours after a phase of increasingly extensive erythroderma. Mycosis fungoides pursues an indolent course with a median survival of eight years. Patients should be managed in a specialised centre by experienced doctors. Treatments include whole body electron beam radiotherapy, topical nitrogen mustard, and photochemotherapy. Systemic treatment with all alkylating drugs and prednisone may be of some benefit and some studies have reported benefit with interferon.[14]

T cell chronic lymphatic leukaemia is a rare variant (2% of this usually B cell disease). It often follows in a rapidly progressive course.

Peripheral T cell lymphomas are a clinically and morphologically heterogeneous group of lymphomas. About 10-20% of all lymphomas are T cell in origin. Peripheral T cell lymphomas are represented in several categories in the working formulation, including diffuse small cleaved cell, diffuse mixed, diffuse large cell, and immunoblastic subtypes. Patients often present with advanced disease. Bone marrow disease, hypercalcaemia, and eosinophilia are relatively common. A poor prognosis has been reported, but this is not universally accepted as other prognostic factors such as age, stage, and performance status were not adjusted for.

The spectrum of T cell lymphomas seen in Japan is similar to that of the peripheral T cell lymphomas described above. Not unexpectedly, these lymphomas are often associated with peripheral adenopathy, hypercalcaemia, and leukaemia. The prognosis is reported to be poor, with early appearance of disease refractory to intensive chemotherapy.

Angioimmunoblastic lymphadenopathy

This abnormal lymphoproliferative disease, although not histologically a malignancy, has a rapidly progressive, often fatal course. Treatment usually consists of high dose prednisone, which should be used to maximum response then tapered. Patients whose condition cannot be maintained without prednisone should have a trial of cyclophosphamide 50-100 mg/m^2 orally every other day, a maintenance immunoregulatory dose which can be continued for long periods if necessary. Many patients with angioimmunoblastic lymphadenopathy develop immunoblastic lymphoma, which if discovered should be treated appropriately.

Conclusion

Although malignant lymphomas are highly treatable, many problems still remain to be addressed in the 1990s. The main topics of interest will be improved treatment and, if possible, cure of advanced stage low grade lymphomas; better identification of patients with intermediate and high grade lymphomas who have a poor prognosis to allow more aggressive and effective treatment; and better management of patients relapsing after first treatment.

1 O'Reilly SE, Connors JM. Non-Hodgkin's lymphoma.I: characterisation and treatment. *BMJ* 1992;**304**:16826.
2 Vose JM, Armitage JO, Weisenburger DD, Bierman PJ, Sorensen S, Hutchins M. The importance of age in survival of patients treated with chemotherapy for aggressive non-Hodgkin's lymphoma. *J Clin Oncol* 1989;**6**:1838-44.
3 O'Reilly SE, Klimo P, Connors JM. Low-dose ACOP-B and VABE: weekly chemotherapy for elderly patients with advanced-stage diffuse large-cell lymphoma. *J Clin Oncol* 1991;**9**:741.
4 O'Reilly SE, Hoskins P, Howdle S, Klasa R, Klimo P, Stuart D, *et al*. POCE chemotherapy—a phase II trial in elderly patients with advanced stage diffuse large cell lymphoma. *Proceedings of the American Society of Clinical Oncology* 1992;**11**:326.
5 Rosengelt F, Rosenberg SA. Diffuse histiocytic lymphoma presenting with gastrointestinal tract lesions. *Cancer* 1980;**45**:2188.
6 Jacobs C, Hoppe RT. Non-Hodgkin's lymphomas of head and neck extranodal sites. *Int J Radiat Oncol Biol Phys* 1985;**11**:357.
7 Cabanillas F, Hagenmeister FB, Bodey GP, Freireich EJ. IMVP-16 an effective regimen for patients with lymphoma who have relapsed after initial combination chemotherapy. *Blood* 1982;**50**:693.
8 Cabanillas F. Experience with salvage regimens at M D Anderson Hospital. *Ann Oncol* 1991;suppl 1,2:31.
9 Velasquez WS, Cabanillas F, Salvador P, McLaughlin P, Fridrik M, Tucker S, *et al*. Effective salvage therapy for lymphoma with cisplatin in combination with high dose Ara-C and dexamethasone (DHAP). *Blood* 1988;**71**:117.
10 Philip T, Armitage J, Spitzer G. High dose therapy and autologous bone marrow transplantation after failure of conventional chemotherapy in adults with intermediate grade of high grade non-Hodgkin's lymphoma. *N Engl J Med* 1987;**24**:316.
11 Coleman CN, Picozzi VJ, Cox RS, McWhirter K, Weis LM, Cohen JR, *et al*. Treatment of lymphoblastic lymphoma in adults. *J Clin Oncol* 1986;**4**:1628.
12 Magrath IT, Janus C, Edwards R, Spiegal R, Jaffe ES, Berard CW, *et al*. An effective therapy for both undifferentiated (including Burkitt's) lymphomas and lymphoblastic lymphomas in children and young adults. *Blood* 1984;**63**:1102-11.
13 Starzl TE, Nalesnik MH, Porter KA, Ho M, Iwatsuki S, Griffith BP, *et al*. Reversibility of lymphomas and lymphoproliferative lesions developing under cyclophosphorin-steroid therapy. *Lancet* 1984;i:583.
14 Weisenburger DD, Sanger WG, Armitage JO. Intermediate lymphocytic lymphoma: immunophenotypic and cytogenic findings. *Blood* 1987;**69**: 1617.
15 Kohn EC, Steis RG, Sausville EA. Phase II trial of intermittent high-dose recombinant interferon alfa-2a in mycosis fungoides and the Sézary syndrome. *J Clin Oncol* 1990;**1**:155-60.

Hodgkin's disease

PATRICE CARDE

The rare disease described in 1832 by Sir Thomas Hodgkin has during the past 30 years been a model for the development of diagnostic and therapeutic procedures. The story starts in 1963 with the claim by Easson that Hodgkin's disease, a type of disseminated cancer, was curable. Several workers showed that if radiotherapy fields were sufficiently large and radiation doses sufficiently high cure was possible. From the beginning an unusual degree of cooperation prevailed between pathologists, radiotherapists, surgeons, radiologists and, later, medical internists and statisticians. From 1957 to 1971 the principles of lymphangiography, surgical staging, clinical staging, pathological classification, isotopic scanning, megavoltage radiation therapy, monochemotherapy, and polychemotherapy were combined in a comprehensive multidisciplinary approach. Statistical analyses, the search for prognostic factors, and controlled trials evolved accordingly.[1] As a consequence survival rose dramatically.

Since the introduction of adjuvant chemotherapy around 1970, however, there has been no evidence of improvement in survival (table I) as documented by the international data bank overview of Hodgkin's disease. The 8671 patients treated from 1970 to 1979 had a similar survival (60% at 20 years) to the 5096 treated after 1980.[2 3] This observation, made in a large cohort of patients treated in expert centres and confirmed in successive cohorts of patients with localised disease during 1972-86, contrasts with the usual optimistic statements.[4 5]

The first reason for the failure to improve survival is the high mortality still associated with Hodgkin's disease in certain groups of patients. A better understanding of the pathogenesis (roles of Epstein-Barr virus, oncogenes, genetics), biological characteristics (lympho-

90

TABLE I—Proportion of patients with Hodgkin's disease achieving complete remission, relapse free survival (in complete responders), and survival at five and 15 years according to Ann Arbor Stage[2]

Clinical stage	No of patients	% With complete remission	% With relapse free survival at five years*	% With relapse free survival at 10 years*	% Survival at 5 years	% Survival at 15 years
I A:						
1970-9	1516	98	80	75	90	70
After 1980	949	98			90	
II A:						
1970-9	2488	95	74	70	88	70
After 1980	1511	94			90	
I B/II B:						
1970-9	1081	87	73	69	80	62
After 1980	721	83			81	
III A:						
1970-9	940	87†	75	63	78	57
After 1980	510	87			83	
III B:						
1970-9	1001	77†	65	61	64	42
After 1980	641	75			70	
IV:						
1970-9	544	62	66	62	54	35
After 1980	752	63			62	

* In complete responders.
† All results for clinical stage III together.

kine production, immunophenotype), and initial prognostic factors of this disease may make the identification of high risk groups easier. Early recognition of the patients in whom treatment is likely to fail or those likely to have a recurrence may provide an opportunity, before irreversible iatrogenic toxicity occurs, to switch to an alternative treatment, with some chances of success.[6]

The second reason for survival not improving is the increasing incidence of deaths that are not related to the disease itself but to the consequences of modern treatments. Patients in the international data bank overview who remained free of disease still had a risk of death more than twice that of a population of the same age and sex. As within six years after diagnosis the risk of dying of unrelated causes overrides that of dying of Hodgkin's disease, and in patients in their early 50s, 20 years after diagnosis the cumulative number of unrelated deaths equals that of deaths from Hodgkin's disease, after 10 years, when virtually no deaths from Hodgkin's disease occur, the standardised mortality ratio is still four to eight times greater in these patients than controls. Less than 5% of these deaths are related to secondary leukaemia or myelodysplasia (for which the causative factor is chemotherapy) or to non-Hodgkin's lymphoma (unknown causes); most of the deaths are from cardiac or pulmonary related diseases (which are caused by radiotherapy, with or without chemotherapy) or secondary solid tumours (due to radiotherapy, immune defects, or chemotherapy).[2 3 7 8] Thus the costs and benefits of chemotherapy and extended field radiotherapy have to be carefully balanced in patients with early stage Hodgkin's disease.

Finally, even though current science may only marginally improve a survival rate as high as 60% at 20 years, it may, and must, urgently improve the quality of patients' lives.[2] The toxicity and stress associated with staging (for instance, by laparotomy, which has no impact on survival), prolonged treatments, and, most of all, gonadal damage and infertility should be quantified and prevented.[9]

Pathology and immunopathology

Both the presence of the Hodgkin and Reed-Sternberg cells and a characteristic cytological environment are required for a pathological diagnosis of Hodgkin's disease. The Rye classification remains the standard. In 5096 cases diagnosed since 1980 in the international data base the proportions of histological subtypes were lymphocyte predominance 6·3%, nodular sclerosis 63·9%, mixed cellularity 24·6%, lymphocyte depletion 1·9%, and unclassified 3·2%.[2] However, morphologically this is an extremely diverse disease.[1]

Recent progress in pathology, immunophenotyping, and cytokine recognition has challenged the concept of Hodgkin's as a single disease. Nodular lymphocyte predominant Hodgkin's disease has been shown to be of a B cell phenotype and to synthesise J chains; high grade B non-Hodgkin's lymphomas evolve commonly from this subtype, which now could be considered a B cell non-Hodgkin's lymphoma. Within the nodular sclerosis category the British National Lymphoma Investigation has described morphologically a more aggressive subtype.[10] Lymphocyte depleted categories of Hodgkin's disease actually represent anaplastic large cell lymphomas exhibiting Ki-1 (CD 30) positivity by morphological and immunological criteria, and some cases of anaplastic non-Hodgkin's lymphoma exhibit all of the features of Hodgkin's disease, including surface receptors for interleukin 9.[12] An admixture of cases of non-Hodgkin's lymphomas with nodular sclerosis lacking mature T or B immunophenotype cannot be distinguished from nodular sclerosis Hodgkin's disease. Cytokine production and histology may be correlated: interleukin 5 receptors and eosinophilic granuloma, secretion of transforming growth factor β in nodular sclerosis Hodgkin's disease.[13 14] Cell lines were also shown to secrete tumour necrosis factor, macrophage colony stimulating factor, and prostaglandin E2. Such correlations may provide clues to the cell of origin of Hodgkin's disease or the prognosis of the disease; they may also help explain the causes of B symptoms; the role of interleukin 1 and interleukin 6 in the pathogenesis of the characteristic fever and correlated sweats has been investigated.[15 16]

Cytogenesis, genetics, and epidemiology

The histopathogenesis of the Reed-Sternberg cell still resists analysis, but there have been some recent insights. Immunophenotyping and genotyping of these cells and derived cell lines, the use of viral probes for the polymerase chain reaction or in situ hybridisation techniques, and results of karyotyping together tentatively indicate a syndrome which fits well with the epidemiology.[12 17 18] Briefly, Reed-Sternberg cells have an immature lymphoid genotype (usually heavy rather than light immunoglobulin gene rearrangements, which are a characteristic of pre-B cell precursors, and T cell receptor gene rearrangements, which are characteristics of pre-T cells). This contrasts with the concomitant phenotypic expression of late "activated" lymphoid cells. The activation markers on these cells (CD 25, CD 30, CDw70, and HLA-DR) are similar to those expressed on Epstein-Barr virus transformed cell lines. This suggests that Reed-Sternberg cells could represent the malignant transformation of immature lymphoid cells that have been infected by the Epstein-Barr virus, a potent activator of lymphoid cells, at the very moment when immunoglobulin or T cell receptor genes are rearranged. Indeed, different techniques have not only shown the presence of the Epstein-Barr virus genome in the cells but have also proved it to be in a clonal form, implying that the virus entered the tumour cells before clonal expansion.[12] In parallel, increased levels of IgG and IgA antibodies against capsid antigens have been recorded, indicating a role for the Epstein-Barr virus during the development of Hodgkin's disease, at least as a cofactor. One possible mechanism is that it acts through a paracrine network of cytokines, mimicking the interaction between the epithelial neoplastic cells and benign lymphoid infiltrating cells seen in nasopharyngeal carcinoma, another cancer related to Epstein-Barr virus.

The lymphocyte predominant category, now considered as a B non-Hodgkin's lymphoma, is set apart; it is probably associated with the evolution of Hodgkin's disease from non-Hodgkin's lymphoma and also with the t(14;18) translocation juxtaposing the BCL2 proto-oncogene, which is implicated in preventing programmed cell death (apoptosis), on to the gene for the Ig heavy chain.

Initial presentation and investigation

The two main histological types of Hodgkin's disease (nodular sclerosis and mixed cellularity) in fact represent two different diseases. The nodular sclerosis type is much more common (70%), occurs at a younger age, and is more common in women; in these cases the nodal disease usually develops at sites related to the drainage of the upper respiratory tract—that is the mediastinum and neck. The mixed cellularity type of disease (30%) more often affects the spleen and the infradiaphragmatic nodes as well as the liver, lung, and bone marrow, presumably by haematogenous spread.[19] Thus staging should be adapted to the histological type as well as to the apparent spread of the disease.

In localised disease the staging (box) has two purposes: firstly, to ensure that the usual locoregional nodal presentation (clinical stages I-II; 60-65% of cases at first diagnosis) represents the actual spread of the disease and thus that limited radiotherapy fields carry a high likelihood of cure; secondly, to estimate through a series of well validated prognostic factors, the potential for the disease to spread outside the radiation fields and therefore the need for adjuvant chemotherapy.[4 20-23] Lymphangiography has proved a more sensitive and specific staging investigation than computed tomography in visualising the retroperineal and iliac node groups in all comparative studies on Hodgkin's disease and should remain central to investigations in localised supradiaphragmatic disease.[24] The risk of splenic disease is highly correlated to positive results on lymphangiography and, therefore, indirectly, it is more sensitive than computed tomography for determining the risk of dissemination through the blood. Unfortunately, lymphangiography, which is time consuming and requires skill and training, tends to be replaced by the easier to perform computed tomography. Biological tests have not all been assessed through large multivariate analyses. Measurement of the

---

Work up recommended in localised supradiaphragmatic presentations

Mandatory	Clinical history and examination
	Ann Arbor or Cotswolds classification
	Blood counts, erythrocyte sedimentation rate, liver function, HIV serology
	Chest radiography, computed tomography of thorax, lymphography (or computed tomography of abdomen and pelvis as second choice)
	Bone marrow biopsy and aspiration
Recommended	Lactate dehydrogenase activity
	Ultrasonography of liver and spleen
Investigational	Computed tomography of abdomen in addition to lymphography
	Magnetic resonance imaging
	Gallium scanning, technetium bone scanning
	Immunoscintigram with antiferritin or antiCD30
	Serum concentrations of soluble CD8, CD25, CD30, IL-6
	Epstein-Barr virus serology

---

erythrocyte sedimentation rate is simple, cheap, well documented, and predicts relapse both initially and during follow up.[20 25-27] Lactate dehydrogenase, which has not been assessed in Hodgkin's disease, and serum concentrations of soluble antigens CD 30, CD 8, CD 25, and interleukin 6 all require multivariate analyses to assess their value.[28]

Staging laparotomy

In localised disease staging laparotomy is no longer required. It was first used to assess the incidence and sites of spread of infradiaphragmatic disease when other tests (including lymphangiography) gave negative results.[29] Up to 62% of patients with supradiaphragmatic stage I-II disease had positive results on laparotomy, which made them pathological stage III-IV.[1 2] This finding explains why in the European Organisation for Research and Treatment of Cancer H1 study more than 50% of patients with mixed cellularity Hodgkin's disease relapsed when radiotherapy alone was given to patients with apparent supradiaphragmatic disease.[30] The clinical presentation was then correlated with the findings of laparotomy.[31 32]

When prophylactic radiotherapy under the diaphragm became routine positive findings at laparotomy, particularly from the spleen, were used as prognostic factors because they correlated with the risk of relapse in patients treated with radiotherapy alone.[21] Patients with positive results were then offered a more intensive treatment (either inverted Y radiotherapy with the drawback of the gonadal irradiation in women, or chemotherapy, or sometimes both). Later, some groups decided not to perform laparotomy at all and to accept a higher relapse rate. By this time it was clear that laparotomy had no impact on survival owing to the efficacy of salvage chemotherapy for patients relapsing after initial radiotherapy.[33] Others decided to omit laparotomy only in patients with poor initial prognostic factors (about 50% chance of survival) since they were due to receive intensive treatment anyway.[4 34 35] Finally, even in the best prognostic group the role of laparotomy has been challenged by the results of a trial in which the type of staging (clinical or laparotomy) was randomised: the six year freedom from progression was only 5% higher in those given laparotomy but paradoxically these patients had a lower survival trend owing to laparotomy related deaths.[4] Furthermore, the emergence of better tolerated and less toxic regimens makes chemotherapy more acceptable, and the associated increase in freedom from progression compensates for the omission of laparotomy. The same is true for patients with stage III disease, in whom down-staging is less of a problem.

Assessment of response

In disseminated disease, when chemotherapy based treatment is indicated, accurate staging of all sites of disease covers two different aims: firstly, to gather prognostic information; secondly, to reassess the same sites after chemotherapy to rule out residual disease. This is required because chemotherapy is less effective at controlling Hodgkin's disease in nodes (around 70% complete response in affected nodes with 30-40% relapse) than is radiotherapy (almost 100% control with rare relapse). Conversely chemotherapy may be superior in visceral disease.

For the same reason much attention has been paid to the early assessment of the response to chemotherapy to identify patients who are very likely to fail, thereby enabling alternative forms of treatment to be started early on, before the patients are overtreated with ineffective but debilitating regimens.[6] Unfortunately, residual masses may contain Hodgkin's disease or only fibrosis, and assessment remains difficult both during and after treatment.[36] Special imaging techniques may help to direct a confirmatory biopsy. Gallium scanning seems to predict reliably a negative biopsy result only in the mediastinum.[37] Nuclear magnetic resonance diagnoses initial marrow disease,[38] but has little to add when treatment has been given or when relapse is suspected. The potential of immunoscintigrams using non-specific antiferritin polyclonal antibodies or specific monoclonal antibodies to the CD 30 determinant needs confirmatory studies.[39]

New staging classification

Implicit to the Ann Arbor classification were the assumptions that early stages of Hodgkin's disease (determined by pathological staging through exploratory laparotomy) should be treated with radiotherapy and that chemotherapy should be reserved for the more advanced cases. The importance of laparotomy diminished with the appearance of newly recognised factors and with the increasing role of chemotherapy in early stage disease. Chemotherapy became more popular because of new, better tolerated regimens and its ability to improve the freedom from progression. Twenty years after formation of the original Ann Arbor classification committee a part of the committee took into account some of these considerations (table II)[40]: hilar disease was separately categorised as a disease site and computed tomography, bulk of the tumour, and assessment of residual disease were included. However, although computed tomography may provide additional information, it cannot replace lymphangiography, and in large multivariate analysis studies there are no data to support the impact of tumour bulk or residual masses.[24] Furthermore, no objective biological test, although some have potential prognostic or follow up importance, has as yet been incorporated to the staging process.

Treatment

The increasing efficacy of treatment of Hodgkin's disease is best reflected by the improvements in relapse free survival which have occurred during the past 20 years, particularly in advanced disease; by contrast survival has improved little.[2]

TABLE II—Cotswolds revision[40] of Ann Arbor staging system

Staging*†	Ann Arbor system	Cotswolds revision
Stage I	1 nodal area or structure—(that is mediastinum=1; thymus=1; Waldeyer's=1; spleen=1)	Same
Stage II	2 or more nodal areas on the same side of the diaphragm	Right and left hilum=1 area each, independent of mediastinum; indicate the No of anatomicalnodal areas affected by a subscript (for example, II₃)
Stage III	At least 1 nodal area on each side of the diaphragm	III1=Upper abdomen (splenic, coeliac, portal) III2=Para-aortic and lower abdomen
Stage IV	Visceral disease	Same
B symptoms	Fever, drenching sweats, weight loss	Same
A	None	Same
E	Extranodal by contiguity, can be included in the nodal radiotherapy field	Same
X		Bulk=mediastinum >1/3 at T5/6; mass >10 cm
CR[u]		Unclear complete remission (residual radiological abnormality)

* Clinical staging without histological confirmation.
† Pathological staging by histological confirmation and eventually surgical exploration (usually laparotomy).

Radiotherapy

Until recently radiotherapy was considered the only treatment with curative potential for disease limited to nodal areas, either localised (stages I-II) or more extensive (stage III).[41] Cure was possible once adequate standards were met concerning the extent of the fields, the dose, and the availability of adequate energy beams.

The contiguous mode of dissemination of Hodgkin's disease along the lymphatic chains accounts for the prolonged restriction of invasion to non-vital areas and for the ability of regional irradiation to cure patients. The technique of extended field radiotherapy proposed by Gilbert as early as 1925 had not been seriously challenged since the first results in a large series by Kaplan in 1962. Extended field techniques treat the next contiguous area, which is thought "likely" to be affected—for example, the mantle and inverted Y fields. Kaplan has shown a dose-response relation for the permanent control of any affected nodal areas.[1] The ideal dose was found to be 40-44 Gy, but dosimetry calculations have shown wide variability in the dose actually received by patients within individual centres. Treatment of all fields daily with fractionation into, at most, five 1·50-2·00 Gy fractions a week is crucial to avoid pulmonary and gastrointestinal radiation injuries. The introduction of adjuvant chemotherapy may have modified the doses required for sterilising affected nodes with ionising radiation. Children, in particular, have benefited from these new approaches, the widespread use of chemotherapy enabling lower radiotherapy doses (20-30 Gy) to be given to affected areas or restricted volumes or both (avoiding the humeral joints, left ventricle, lungs, etc) so that subsequent abnormalities in growth and function are limited.[42] Technical advances (computed tomography, treatment planning, field simulation, portal imaging, custom contoured cerro-bend blocks, opposed field techniques, field modification during treatment, and quality assurance programmes) have made it possible to deliver high radiation doses (6·25 MeV linear accelerator photons) to deep tissues while sparing unaffected superficial tissues. Further developments have allowed superficial treatments with limited pene-tration (electron beams from linear accelerators).[43]

Chemotherapy

The efficacy of chemotherapy can be assessed more easily in advanced Hodgkin's disease (stages IIIB-IV), than in localised disease because chemotherapy repre-sents the main treatment and relapses are frequent. Three main chemotherapy regimens have been tested: MOPP (mustine, vincristine, procarbazine, and prednisolone), AVBD (doxorubicin, bleomycin, vinblastine, and dacarbazine), and a combination of both (tables III and IV). MOPP, the standard chemo-therapy, alternates two week cycles of treatment (intravenous and oral) with rest periods, which allow recovery from the serious toxicity usually experienced.[54] Adequate dosing has an impact on the results,[55] and usually not more than eight cycles need to be given. Derivatives of MOPP may be better tolerated, particularly when mustine is replaced by chlorambucil.[46] Cures with ABVD in patients who have relapsed after treatment with MOPP provided evidence that salvage with chemotherapy could be achieved in patients in whom a first induction regimen failed.[56] Only the Cancer and Leukaemia Group B (CALGB) directly compared MOPP and ABVD in advanced Hodgkin's disease. Its study showed a significantly higher relapse free survival with ABVD.[45] This finding was confirmed when ABVD was compared with MOPP in patients also receiving radiotherapy for localised Hodgkin's disease.[4 47 57]

TABLE III — Main chemotherapy regimens for Hodgkin's disease

Drugs	Dose (mg/m²)	Route	Scheme	Regimen
MOPP:				
Mustine	6	Intravenous	1 and 8	28 Day cycle—2 weeks' treatment,
Vincristine	1·4	Intravenous	1 and 8	2 weeks' rest.
Procarbazine	100	Oral	1 to 14	6 Cycles for adjuvant treatment
Prednisolone	40	Oral	1 to 14	and 6-12 for therapeutic
ABVD:				
Doxorubicin	25	Intravenous	1 and 15	28 Day treatment cycle
Bleomycin	10	Intravenous	1 and 15	6 Cycles for adjuvant treatment
Vinblastine	6	Intravenous	1 and 15	and 6-12 for therapeutic
Dacarbazine	375	Intravenous	1 and 15	
MOPP/ABV:				
MOPP 1 week plus			1 to 7	28 Day cycle—2 weeks' treatment
Doxorubicin	35	Intravenous	Day 8	and 2 weeks' rest.
Bleomycin	10	Intravenous	Day 8	6 Cycles for adjuvant treatment
Vinblastine	6	Intravenous	Day 8	and 6-12 for therapeutic
Prednisone	40	Oral	8-14	
EBVP:				
Epirubicin	75	Intravenous	Day 1	21 Day treatment cycle
Bleomycin	6	Intravenous	Day 1	6 Cycles for adjuvant treatment
Vinblastine	6	Intravenous	Day 1	
Prednisone	40	Oral	1 to 5	
VBM:				
Vinblastine	6	Intravenous	1 and 8	28 Day cycle—2 weeks' treatment
Bleomycin	10	Intravenous	1 and 8	and 2 weeks' rest.
Methotrexate	30	Intravenous	1 and 8	6 Cycles for adjuvant treatment
CEP:				
Lomustine	80	Oral	Day 1	28 to 46 day cycle
Etoposide	100	Oral	Day 1 to 5	6-8 Cycles for salvage treatment
Prednimustine	60	Oral	Day 1 to 5	

In EBVP, a popular ABVD derivative, in which epirubicin has been substituted for doxorubicin; dacarbazine was dropped from the regimen because of its equivocal efficacy and serious gastrointestinal toxicity.[58]

A benefit was expected from the combination of MOPP and a derivative of ABVD.[49] The superiority of the combination over MOPP alone was confirmed by the European Organisation for Research and Treatment of Cancer and the CALGB trial.[6 45] The mechanism underlying the combination's greater effect was investigated by the CALGB trial by adding a third arm—ABVD alone—and by the Société Française d'Oncologie Pediatrique trial in children: the combination was not superior to ABVD alone, suggesting that ABVD is intrinsically more efficient than MOPP. This hypothesis is supported by the design of the CALGB trial, in which an unbalanced

TABLE IV — Main chemotherapy results in Hodgkin's disease

Regimen	No of patients (stage)	% In complete remission	% With relapse free survival (in complete remission)	% With freedom from progression (all)	% Survival (all)	Remarks
MOPP and derived:						
MOPP[44]	188 (III-IV)	84	66 at 14 years	54 at 14 years	48 at 14 years	Unmatched, phase II trial
MOPP[47,49]	114 (IIB-III)	81	77 at 7 years	63 at 7 years	68 at 7 years	v ABVD (+radiotherapy)
MOPP[48]	43 (IV)	74	44 at 7 years	35 at 7 years	61 at 7 years	v MOPP/ABVD
MOPP[6]	95 (III-IV)	60	65 at 4 years	49 at 4 years	62 at 4 years	v MOPP/ABVD
MOPP[45]	400/3 (III-IV)	72	48 at 5 years		79 at 5 years	6 Cycles of MOPP v 12 of MOPP/ABVD v 6 of ABVD
ChlVPP[46]	229 (II-IV)	85	71 at 10 years		65 at 10 years	Better tolerated than MOPP
ABVD regimen:						
ABVD[47,49]	118 (IIB-III)	92	88 at 7 years	81 at 7 years		v MOPP (+radiotherapy)
ABVD[45]	400/3 (IIB-III)	88	60 at 5 years		77 at 7 years	6 Cycles v 12 of MOPP+ABVD v 6 of MOPP
Alternating regimens:						
MOPP/ABVD[48]	45 (IV)	89	77 at 7 years	68 at 7 years	82 at 7 years	v MOPP
MOPP/ABVD[49]	152 (IIB-IV)	88	72 at 5 years	65 at 5 years	81 at 5 years	v half MOPP+half ABVD (+radiotherapy) v MOPP
MOPP/ABVD[46]	95 (IIIB-IV)	61	64 at 4 years	72 at 4 years	75 at 4 years	12 Cycles v 6 of MOPP v 6 of ABVD
MOPP/ABVD[45]	400/3 (III-IV)	83	65 at 5 years		79 at 5 years	v 8 cycles of MOPP/ABVD (+radiotherapy)
MOPP/ABV[50]	146 (IIIB-IV)	85	75 at 4 years		84 at 4 years	v 8 cycles of hybrid MOPP/ABV
MOPP/ABVD[50]	141 (III-IV)	82	70 at 4 years		84 at 4 years	(+radiotherapy) Phase II trial
MOPP/ABV[51]	170 (II-IV)			65 at 7 years	80 at 7 years	v MOPP/ABVB (+radiotherapy)
half MOPP/ half ABVD[49]	148 (IIB-IV)	88	78 at 5 years	70 at 5 years	80 at 5 years	
New adjuvant regimens:						
EBVP[52]	64 (I-IIIA)	97			92 at 3·5 years	Experienced in >300 patients (+radiotherapy)
VBM[53,71]	26 (I-II)	100	100 at 5 years	100 at 5 years	100 at 5 years	Small series; bleomycin tapered (+radiotherapy)

MOPP = Mustine, vincristine, procarbazine, and prednisolone.
ChlVPP = Chlorambucil, vincristine, procarbazine, and prednisolone.
ABVD = Doxorubicin, bleomycin, vinblastine, and prednisolone.

Treatment that may result in delayed death after Hodgkin's disease

Treatment	Possible adverse effects
Laparotomy	Embolism and sepsis and perhaps secondary leukaemia and solid tumours[4 8]
Nitrogen mustard, other alkylating drugs, etoposide	Secondary leukaemia[61 62]
Bleomycin plus mediastinal irradiation	Lung fibrosis
Radiotherapy of left ventricle	Cardiac complications in young patients[4 8 60]

---

number of cycles (12 of MOPP/ABVD v six of ABVD) may have favoured the combination.[45] The assessment of new ABVD derivatives should therefore be given the highest priority.

Prevention of lethal toxicity

Only recently has it been appreciated that treatment related toxicity has jeopardised long term survival in substantial proportions of patients.[7 8 59] The relative risk of death in patients cured of Hodgkin's disease was over three times that in the general population in the European series.[59] In the international data base series only 6% of the deaths in patients without evidence of active Hodgkin's disease were recorded as treatment related, with these deaths occurring mostly in the first 10 years.[7] However, treatment probably contributed to many of the deaths attributed to an unspecified cause (3%), intercurrent disease (14%), and secondary cancer (10%).[2] The box lists the potentially lethal factors that can be avoided.

It seems likely that the current and fashionable introduction of more intense treatments (high dose chemotherapy or radiotherapy, or both, before autologous marrow or peripheral stem cell transplantations) in large cohorts of patients (supposedly at high risk or as a "consolidation" measure) will cause a significant incidence of delayed death in 10 years' time. Similarly, inhibitors of topoisomerase II (such as etoposide) have recently been increasingly used; these may be responsible for secondary leukaemias associated with balanced translocations.[61] Finally, radiotherapy is probably responsible for most of the secondary solid tumours: reduced field sizes and possibly dose tapering should be explored.[7 62]

Assessment and prevention of delayed morbidity

No sufficiently sensitive tests are at present available to allow monitoring of cardiac and pulmonary risks; this is shown by the disappearance after two years of follow up of initial differences between patients treated with mantle irradiation plus MOPP or ABVD.[4] However, long term follow up of cohorts of patients treated with heart irradiation or anthracyclines, or both, may show persisting effects, as seen recently in children. This issue is being investigated.[8] Efforts are underway to select the least toxic regimens or to investigate the possibility of using drugs with a potentially cardioprotective effect—for example, free radical scavengers or the ferrous chelator razoxane 187.[63]

Unfortunately, gonadal toxicity has rarely been monitored accurately in either sex and few efforts have been made to avoid the alkylating drugs responsible for this problem. Gonadal protection from radiotherapy has also been suboptimal, and few of the potential protectors are being tested.[64] Sperm storage is not offered to all patients, indicating that medical staff are not well informed.

These issues are particularly important in children, where the freedom from progression and survival figures are generally better than those observed in adults. In children chemotherapy alone remains a valid option owing to the problems with growth associated with radiotherapy. Gonadotoxicity and leukaemogenicity remain problems, despite which alkylating drugs are still widely used.[65] The risk of long term toxicity, including cardiac and gonadal damage, should increasingly influence the choice of drugs.

New approaches to early stage disease

The use of different historical databases may explain why no consensus has emerged for treating localised supradiaphragmatic Hodgkin's disease.[66 67] Only prominent general recommendations are possible in reference to recent and ongoing clinical trials: for example, staging laparotomy is not necessary, stratification to tailor both investigation and treatment to pretreatment characteristics should avoid undertreatment and overtreatment, and prolonged follow up is essential to identify delayed toxicities. Since few events occur in early stage disease attempts to establish prognostic groups and indexes must rely on large cohorts of patients with prospectively registered initial characteristics and must take into account the type of staging and treatment used. Some prognostic factors are simple enough to be of practical help: systemic (B) symptoms, erythrocyte sedimentation rate, tumour bulk expressed as the number of nodal sites affected or as the size of the mediastinal mass, and older age.[22 25 68]

A practical strategy to adjust treatment intensity to likely response might be one recognising four prognostic groups arbitrarily separated. In the very favourable group (for instance, stage I lymphocyte predominant Hodgkin's disease affecting high cervical nodes in women) the only treatment necessary may be supradiaphragmatic radiotherapy. In favourable patients and even in unselected patients who have not had a laparotomy subtotal nodal irradiation is acceptable.[35 43 66 67 69] In such patients adjuvant vinblastine used alone provided a persisting advantage in freedom from progression without an increase in secondary leukaemias.[70] This observation supports the use of low toxic adjuvant regimens such as the VBM (vinblastine, bleomycin, and methotrexate) or EBVP in such cases.[58 71] One study found that chemotherapy alone provided equivalent results to chemotherapy and radiotherapy in favourable patients but inferior results in unfavourable patients.[72] In unfavourable patients most randomised trials have shown superior freedom from progression with combined chemotherapy and radiotherapy to that with radiotherapy alone, though a survival advantage has not been shown.[22 66] Meta-analyses are being conducted to investigate this question on a broader database. Adjuvant ABVD has proved better than MOPP in all available randomised trials.[4 57] Finally, a very unfavourable group has not yet been satisfactorily defined. For patients with large mediastinal masses, who clearly belong to this group, both radiotherapy alone and MOPP alone are suboptimal,[73-76] making comparisons of chemotherapy alone with radiotherapy alone less attractive. The two trials which compared MOPP alone with radiotherapy alone provided contradictory results.[75 76]

Older age is the most adverse prognostic factor, although age has not been proved to be associated with a more aggressive disease pattern. Ways to deliver more effective chemotherapy and radiotherapy in patients over 65 are being investigated.

Marrow transplantation

The reported efficacy of any salvage chemotherapy regimen must take into account the case mix, in particular, both the time to relapse and the type of chemotherapy previously administered. For failure of treatment with MOPP and its derivatives the best results to date (20% freedom from progression at five years) have been reported with ABVD.[56] Conversely, MOPP has proved less effective in patients in whom ABVD had failed.[49] After sequential or alternating MOPP/ABVD few conventional dose salvage regimens have proved effective. The best results have been reported with the CEP (CCNU (lomustine), etoposide, and prednimustine) regimen (47% rate of complete remission with 20% survival at five years).[77] Monochemotherapy may offer valuable palliation in those patients in whom salvage chemotherapy fails and who are not eligible for high dose chemotherapy.[78]

High dose chemotherapy — for instance, CBV (cyclophosphamide, carmustine, etoposide) followed by autologous bone marrow transplantation[79] — is an alternative approach. In one study complete remission and three year survival rates over 50% and 30% respectively were reported in heavily pretreated patients.[79] However, lethal toxicities do occur with this approach (in 17% of patients in the large European autologous bone marrow transplantation series).[80] Patients unsuitable for transplantation include those in whom complete remission has never been achieved, those who have had previous extensive irradiation, or, in some centres, those in a second complete remission. The overall impact of autologous bone marrow transplantation is unknown as patients treated with this method are usually highly selected for the procedure.[80] The use of peripheral blood stem cells and growth factors in addition to or in place of autologous marrow may help haematological tolerance.[81 82] Several European trials are now randomising bone marrow transplantation and conventional chemotherapy in well defined patients with relapse after in field radiotherapy or after MOPP plus ABVD or an equivalent regimen. Long term toxicities have yet to be well quantified.[80] The procedure should not at this time be extended to patients who could be cured by other methods — that is, initially high risk patients who achieved a first remission and those with relapse after radiotherapy alone or radiotherapy combined with less intensive chemotherapy regimens.

Conclusion

The Cotswold revision of the staging classification should help to

105

improve the management of Hodgkin's disease. Objective biological parameters need to be identified that can be used to predict the progression of the disease. These may emerge from the recent advances in knowledge of the disease's aetiology and pathogenesis. Broad data banks like that of the international data base overview should improve assessment of the likely prognosis with treatment strategies of different severities. With these developments and the increased use of adjuvant chemotherapy staging laparotomy may no longer be used.

The apparent advantage of combined radiotherapy and chemotherapy over either treatment alone in early stage disease may be confirmed by ongoing meta-analyses. New approaches to early stage disease that combine low dose radiotherapy with non-toxic chemotherapy in an attempt to decrease the high death rate related to treatment seem more important. Although most of the drugs responsible for secondary leukaemia have been recognised (mustine, nitrosoureas, and etoposide), they are still included in regimens given to children and their use has not been restricted to high risk patients. That radiotherapy causes secondary solid tumours is well recognised, but the cardiovascular consequences of mediastinal irradiation are probably underestimated. Recent results from large randomised trials confirm that large patient cohorts, multicentre studies, and long term follow up are needed to improve the management of patients. The advances in treatment of Hodgkin's disease should benefit the entire specialty of oncology.

1 Kaplan HS. *Hodgkin's disease*. Cambridge, Massachusetts: Harvard University, 1980.
2 Somers R, Henry-Amar M, Meerwaldt JH, Carde P, eds. *Treatment strategy in Hodgkin's disease*. London, Paris: INSERM/John Libbey Eurotext, 1990. (Colloque INSERM No 196.)
3 Henry-Amar M, Somers R. Survival outcome after Hodgkin's disease: a report from the international data base on Hodgkin's disease. *Sem Oncol* 1990;17: 758-68.
4 Carde P, Hagenbeek A, Hayat M, Monconduit M, Thomas J, Burgers MJV, et al. Clinical staging versus laparotomy and combined modality with MOPP versus ABVD in early stage Hodgkin's disease: the H6 twin randomized trials from the EORTC lymphoma cooperative group 1992 (in press).
5 Urba WJ, Longo DL. Hodgkin's disease. *N Engl J Med* 1992;326:678-87.
6 Somers R, Henry-Amar M, Carde P, Najman A. MOPP vs alternating 2 MOPP/2 ABVD in advanced Hodgkin's disease (HD). *Proceedings of the American Society of Clinical Oncology* 1988;914:236.
7 Henry-Amar M, Hayat M, Meerwaldt JH, Burgers M, Carde P, Somers R, et al. Causes of death after therapy for early stage Hodgkin's disease entered on EORTC protocols. *Int J Radiat Oncol Biol Phys* 1990;19:1155-7.
8 Hohl RJ, Schilsky RL, Non malignant complications of therapy for Hodgkin's disease. *Hematol Oncol Clin North Am* 1989;3(2):331-43.
9 Fobair P, Hoppe RT, Bloom J, Cox R, Vanghese A, Spiegel D. Psychosocial problems among survivors of Hodgkin's disease. *J Clin Oncol* 1986;4: 805-14.

10 McLennan KA, Bennett MH, Tu A, Vaughan Hudson B, Easterling MJ, Vaughan Hudson G, et al. Relationship of histopathologic features to survival and relapse in nodular sclerosing Hodgkin's disease: a study of 1659 patients. Cancer 1989;64:1686-93.

11 Culine S, Henry-Amar M, Diebold J, Audebert A, Chomette G, Prudhomme de Saint-Maur P, et al. Relationship of histological subtypes to prognosis in early stage Hodgkin's disease: a review of 312 cases in a controlled clinical trial. Eur J Cancer 1989;25:551-6.

12 Stein H, Herbst H, Anagnostopoulos I, Niedobitek G, Dallenbach F, Kratzsch HC. The nature of Hodgkin and Reed-Sternberg cells, their association with EBV, and their relationship to anaplastic large-cell lymphoma. Annals of Oncology 1991;2:33-8.

13 Samoszuk M, Nansen L. Detection of interleukin-5 messenger RNA in Reed-Sternberg cells of Hodgkin's disease with eosinophilia. Blood 1990;75:13-6.

14 Kadin ME, Agnarsson BA, Ellingsworth LR, Newcom SR. Immunohistochemical evidence of a role for transforming growth factor beta in the pathogenesis of nodular sclerosing hodgkin's disease. Am J Pathol 1990;136: 1209-14.

15 Ree HJ, Crowley JP, Dinarello CA. Anti-interleukin-1 reactive cells in Hodgkin's disease. Cancer 1987;59:1717-20.

16 Jücker M, Abts H, Li W, Schindler R, Merz H, Günther A, et al. Expression of interleukin-6 and interleukin-6 receptor in Hodgkin's disease. Blood 1991;77:2413-8.

17 Diehl V, Von Kalle C, Fonatsch C, Tesch H, Jücker M, Schaadt M. The cell of origin in Hodgkin's disease. Sem Oncol 1990;17:660-72.

18 Mueller N. An epidemiologist's view of the new molecular biology findings in Hodgkin's disease. Annals of Oncology 1991;2:23-8.

19 Tubiana M, Hayat M, Henry-Amar M, Breur K, Van Der Werf-Messing B, et al. Five year results of the EORTC randomized study of splenectomy and spleen irradiation in clinical stages I and II of Hodgkin's disease. Eur J Cancer 1981;17:355-63.

20 Tubiana M, Henry-Amar M, Van Der Werf-Messing B, Henry J, Abbatucci J, Burgers M, et al. A multivariate analysis of prognostic factors in early stages Hodgkin's disease. Int J Rad Oncol Biol Phys 1985;11:23-30.

21 Mauch BP, Tarbell N, Weinstein H, Silver B, Goffman T, Osteen R, et al. Stage IA and IIA supradiaphragmatic Hodgkin's disease: prognostic factors in surgically staged patients treated with mantle and paraaortic irradiation J Clin Oncol 1988;6(10):1576-83.

22 Tubiana M, Henry-Amar M, Carde P, Burgers JMV, Hayat M, Van Der Schueren E, et al. Toward comprehensive management tailored to prognostic factors of patients with clinical stages I and II in Hodgkin's disease. The EORTC Lymphoma Group controlled clinical trials: 1964-1987. Blood 1989;73:47-56.

23 Specht L. Prognostic factors in Hodgkin's disease. Cancer Treat Rev 1991;18:21-53.

24 Mansfield CM, Fabian C, Jones S, Van Slyck EJ, Grogea P, Morrison F, et al. Comparison of lymphangiography and computed tomography scanning in evaluating abdominal disease in stages III and IV Hodgkin's disease. Cancer 1990;66:2295-9.

25 Haybittle JL, Hayhoe FG, Easterling MJ, Jelliffe AM, Bennett MH, Vaughan Hudson G, et al. Review of British National lymphoma investigation of Hodgkin's disease and development of prognostic index. Lancet 1985;i: 967-72.

26 Henry-Amar M, Friedman S, Hayat M, Somers R, Meerwaldt JH, Carde P, et al. Erythrocyte sedimentation rate predicts early relapse and survival in early-stage Hodgkin disease. Ann Intern Med 1991;114:361-5.

27 Friedman S, Henry-Amar M, Cosset JM, Carde P, Hayat M, Dupouy N, et al. Evolution of erythrocyte sedimentation rate as predictor of early relapse in posttherapy early-stage Hodgkin's disease. J Clin Oncol 1988;6:596-602.

28 Gause A, Pohl C, Tschiersch A, Da Costa L, Jung W, Diehl V, et al. Clinical significance of soluble CD30 antigen in the sera of patients with untreated Hodgkin's disease. Blood 1991;77:1983-8.

29 Glatstein E, Guernsey JM, Rosenberg SA. The value of laparotomy and splenectomy in the staging of Hodgkin's disease. Cancer 1969;24:709-18.

30 Tubiana M, Henry-Amar M, Hayat M, Breur K, Van Der Werf-Messing B, Burgers M, et al. Long-term results of the EORTC randomized study of irradiation and vinblastine in clinical stages I and II of Hodgkin's disease. Euro J Cancer 1979;15:645-57.

31 Tubiana M, Henry-Amar M, Hayat M, Burgers M, Qasim M, Somers R, et al. The EORTC treatment of early stages of Hodgkin's disease: the role of radiotherapy. Int J Rad Oncol Biol Phys 1984;10:197-210.

32 Brada M, Easton DF, Horwich A, Peckham MJ. Clinical presentation as a predictor of laparotomy findings in supradiaphragmatic stage I and II Hodgkin's disease. Radiother Oncol 1986;5:15-22.

33 Bergsagel DE, Alison RE, Bean HA, Brown TC, Bush RS, Clark RM, *et al.* Results of treating Hodgkin's disease without a policy of laparotomy staging. *Cancer Treatment Reports* 1982;**66**:717-31.

34 Carde P, Hayat M, Cosset JM, Somers R, Burgers JMV, Sizoo W, *et al.* Comparison of total nodal irradiation versus combined sequence of mantle irradiation with mechlorethamine, vincristine, procarbazine, and prednisone in clinical stages I and II Hodgkin's disease: experience of the European Organization for Research and Treatment of Cancer. *National Cancer Institute Monographs* 1988;**6**:303-10.

35 Carde P, Burgers JMV, Henry-Amar M, Hayat M, Sizoo W, Van Der Schueren E, *et al.* Clinical stages I and II Hodgkin's disease: a specifically tailored therapy according to prognostic factors. *J Clin Oncol* 1988;**6**: 239-52.

36 Radford JA, Cowan RA, Flanagan M, Dunn G, Crowther D, Johnson RJ, *et al.* The significance of residual mediastinal abnormality on the chest radiograph following treatment for Hodgkin's disease. *J Clin Oncol* 1988;**6**:940-6.

37 Hagemeister FB, Fesus SM, Lamki LM, Haynie TP. Role of the gallium scan in Hodgkin's disease. *Cancer* 1990;**65**:1090-6.

38 Smith SR, Williams CE, Edwards RHT, Davies JN. Quantitative magnetic resonance studies of lumbar vertebral marrow in patients with refractory or relapsed Hodgkin's disease. *Ann Oncol* 1991;**2**:39-42.

39 Carde P, Pfreundschuh M, Da Costa L, Manil L, Lumbroso JD, Caillou B, *et al. Recent results cancer Res* 1989;**117**:101-11.

40 Lister TA, Crowther D, Sutcliffe SB, Glatstein F, Canellos GP, Young RC, *et al.* Report of a committee convened to discuss the evaluation and staging of patients with Hodgkin's disease: Cotswolds meeting. *J Clin Oncol* 1989;**7**: 1630-6.

41 Peckham MJ, Ford HT, McElwain JT, Harmer CL, Atkinson K, Austin DE. The results of radiotherapy for Hodgkin's disease. *Br J Cancer* 1975;**32**: 391-400.

42 Dionet C, Oberlin O, Habrand JL, Vilcoq J, Madelain M, Dutou L, *et al.* Initial chemotherapy and low-dose radiation in limited fields in childhood Hodgkin's disease: result of a joint cooperative study by the French Society of Pediatric Oncology (SFOP) and Hôpital Saint-Louis, Paris. *Int J Radiat Oncol Biol Phys* 1988;**15**:341-6.

43 Hoppe RT. Radiation therapy in the management of Hodgkin's disease. *Sem Oncol* 1990;**17**: 704-15.

44 Longo DL, Young RC, Wesley M, Hubbard SM, Duffey PL, Jaffe EE, *et al.* 20 Years of MOPP therapy for Hodgkin's disease. *J Clin Oncol* 1986;**4**: 1296-306.

45 Cannellos GP, Propert K, Cooper R, Nissen N, Anderson J, Antman KH, *et al.* MOPP vs ABVD vs MOPP alternating with ABVB in advanced Hodgkin's disease: a prospective randomised CALGB trial. *Proceedings of the American Society of Oncology* 1988;**8**:230.

46 Selby P, Patel P, Milan S, Meldrum M, Mansi J, Mbidde E, *et al.* ChlVPP combination chemotherapy for Hodgkin's disease: long term results. *Br J Canc* 1990;**62**:279-85.

47 Santoro A, Viviani S, Zucali R, Ragni G, Bonfante V, Valagussa P, *et al.* Comparative results and toxicity of MOPP vs AVBD combined with radiotherapy (RT) in PSIIB, III (A, B) Hodgkin's disease (HD). [Abstract]. Proceedings of the American Society of Oncology 1983;**2**:223.

48 Bonadonna G, Santoro A, Valagussa P, Viviani S, Zucali R, Bonfante V, *et al.* Current status of the Milan trials for Hodgkin's disease in adults. In: Cavalli F, Bonadonna G, Rosencweig M, eds. *Proceedings of the second international conference on malignant lymphomas, Lugano, June 13-14, 1984.* Boston: Martinus Nijhoff Publishing, 1985:299-307.

49 Bonadonna G, Santoro A, Gianni AM, Viviani S, Siena S, Gregni M, *et al.* Primary and salvage chemotherapy in advanced Hodgkin's disease: the Milan Cancer Institute experience. *Ann Oncol* 1991;**1**:9-16.

50 Connors JM, Klimo P, Adams G, Burns B, Cooper I, Meyer R, *et al.* MOPP/ABV hybrid versus alternating MOPP/ABVD for advanced Hodgkin's disease. *Proceedings of the American Society of Clinical Oncology* 1992;**11**:317.

51 O'Reilly SE, Hoskins P, Klimo P, Connors JM. MACOP-B and VACOP-B in diffuse large cell lymphoma and MOPP/ABV in Hodgkin's disease. *Ann Oncol* 1991;**2**(suppl 1):17-23.

52 Zittoun R, Eghbali H, Audebert A, Rojouan J, David B, Blank CM, *et al.* Association d'epirubicine, bleomycine, vinblastine, et prednisone (EPVB) avant radiotherapie dans les stades localisés de la maladie de Hodgkin. Essai de phase II. *Bull Canc* 1987;**74**:1515-7.

53 Hoppe RT, Horning SJ, Hancock SL, Rosenberg SA. Current Stanford clinical trials for Hodgkin's disease. *Recent Results Cancer Res* 1989;**117**: 182-90.

54 De Vita VT, Serpick AA, Carbone PP. Combination chemotherapy in the treatment of advanced Hodgkin's disease. *Ann Intern Med* 1970;**73**:891-5.

55 Carde P, Mackintosh FR, Rosenberg SA. A dose and time response analysis of the treatment of Hodgkin's disease with MOPP chemotherapy. *J Clin Oncol* 1983;**1**:146-53.
56 Santoro A, Bonfante V, Bonadonna G. Salvage chemotherapy with ABVD in MOPP-resistant Hodgkin's disease. *Ann Intern Med* 1982;**96**:139-43.
57 Santoro A, Bonadonna G, Valagussa P, Zucali R, Viviani S, Villani F, *et al*. Long-term results of combined chemotherapy-radiotherapy approach in Hodgkin's disease: superiority of ABVD plus radiotherapy versus MOPP plus radiotherapy. *J Clin Oncol* 1987;**5**:27-37.
58 Hoerni B, Orgerie MB, Eghbali H. Nouvelle association d'épirubicine, bléomycine, vinblastine et prednisone (EBVP II) avant radiothérapie dans les stades localisés de maladie de Hodgkin. Essai de phase II chez 50 malades. *Bull Cancer* 1990;**75**:789-94.
59 Cosset JM, Henry-Amar M, Meerwaldt JH. Long-term toxicity of early stages of Hodgkin's disease therapy: the EORTC experience. *Ann Oncol* 1991;**2**: 7782.
60 Cosset JM, Henry-Amar M, Pellae-Cosset B, Carde P, Girinski T, Tubiana M, *et al*. Pericarditis and myocardial infarctions after Hodgkin's disease therapy at the Institut Gustave Roussy. *Int J Radiat Oncol Biol Phys* 1990;**21**:447-9.
61 Ratain MJ, Rowley JD. Therapy-related acute myeloid leukemia secondary to inhibitors of topoisomerase II: from the bedside to the target genes. *Ann Oncol* 1992;**3**:107-11.
62 Tucker MA, Coleman CN, Cox RS, Varghese A, Rosenberg SA. Risk of second cancers after treatment for Hodgkin's disease. *N Engl J Med* 1988;**318**:76-81.
63 Speyer JL, Green MD, Zeleniuch-Jacquotte A, Wernz JC, Rey M, Sanger J, *et al*. ICRF-187 permits longer treatment with doxorubicin in women with breast cancer. *J Clin Oncol* 1992;**10**:117-27.
64 Jégou B, Velez de la Calle JF, Bauché F. Protective effect of medroxyprogesterone acetate plus testosterone against radiation-induced damage to the reproductive function of male rats and their offspring. *Proc Natl Acad Sci USA* 1991;**88**:8710-4.
65 Ekert H, Waters KD, Smith PJ, Toogood I, Mauger D. Treatment with MOPP or ChlVPP chemotherapy only for all stages of childhood Hodgkin's disease. *J Clin Oncol* 1988;**6**: 845-50.
66 Rosenberg SA, Kaplan HS: The evolution and summary results of the Stanford randomized clinical trials of the management of Hodgkin's disease: 19621984. *Int J Radiat Oncol Biol Phys* 1985;**11**:5-32.
67 Horwich A. The management of early Hodgkin's Disease. *Blood* 1990;**4**: 181-6.
68 Specht L. Prognostic factors in Hodgkin's disease. *Cancer Treat Rev* 1991;**18**:2153.
69 Mauch BP, Tarbell N, Weinstein H, Silver S, Goffman T, Osteen R, *et al*. Stage IA and IIA supradiaphragmatic Hodgkin's disease: prognostic factors in surgically staged patients treated with mantle and paraaortic irradiation. *J Clin Oncol* 1988;**6**:1576-83.
70 Carde P, Henry-Amar M, Tubiana M, Van Der Werf-Messing B, Henry J, Abbatucci J, *et al*. No increased incidence of second leukemias in patients treated with vinblastine alone or associated with procarbazine following radiotherapy in 2 successive EORTC controlled trials (1964-1976) in clinical stages I-II Hodgkin's disease. *Proceedings of the American Society of Clinical Oncology* 1985;**4**:212.
71 Horning SJ, Hoppe RT, Hancock SL, Rosenberg SA. Vinblastine, bleomycin and methotrexate: an effective adjuvant in favorable Hodgkin's disease. *J Clin Oncol* 1988;**6**:1822-31.
72 Pavlovsky S, Maschio M, Santarelli MT, Muriel FS, Corrado C, Garcia I, *et al*. Randomized trial of chemotherapy versus chemotherapy plus radiotherapy for stage I-II Hodgkin's disease. *J Natl Cancer Inst* 1988;**80**:1466-73.
73 Cosset JM, Henry-Amar M, Carde P, Clarke D, Lebourgeois JP, Tubiana M. The prognostic significance of large mediastinal masses in the treatment of Hodgkin's disease. The experience of the Institut Gustave-Roussy. *Hematol Oncol* 1984;**2**:33-43.
74 Longo DL, Russo A, Duffey PL, Hubbard SM, Glatstein E, Hill JB, *et al*. Treatment of advanced-stage massive mediastinal Hodgkin's disease: the case for combined modality treatment. *J Clin Oncol* 1991;**9**:227-35.
75 Longo DL, Glatstein E, Duffey PL, Young RC, Hubbard SM, Urba WJ, *et al*. Radiation therapy versus combination chemotherapy in the treatment of early-stage Hodgkin's disease: seven-year results of a prospective randomized trial. *J Clin Oncol* 1991;**9**:906-17.
76 Cimino G, Biti GP, Anselmo AP, Enrici RM, Bellesi GP, Bosi A, *et al*. MOPP chemotherapy versus extended-field radiotherapy in the management of pathological stages I-IIA Hodgkin's disease. *J Clin Oncol* 1989;**7**:732-7.
77 Bonadonna G, Valgussa P, Santoro A. Prognosis of Hodgkin's disease treated with chemotherapy alone or combined with radiotherapy. *Cancer Surv* 1985;**4**:439-58.
78 Mead GM, Harker WG, Kushlan P, Rosenberg SA. Single agent palliative chemotherapy for end-stage Hodgkin's disease. *Cancer* 1982;**50**:829-35.

79 Jaganath S, Dicke KA, Armitage JO, Cabanillas FF, Horwitz LJ, Vellekoop L, *et al*. High dose cyclophosphamide carmustine and epotoside and autologous bone marrow transplantation for relapsed Hodgkin's disease. *Ann Intern Med* 1986;**104**:163-8.

80 Goldstone AH, Linch DC. Bone marrow transplantation in the malignant lymphomas. *Recent advances in haematology* 1992;**6**:14971.

81 Kessinger A, Armitage JO, Smith DM, Landmark JD, Bierman PJ, Weisenburger DD. High dose therapy and autologous peripheral blood stem cell transplantation for patients with lymphoma. *Blood* 1989;**74**:1260-5.

82 Nemunaitis J, Rabinowe SN, Singer JW, Bierman PJ, Vose JM, Freedman AS, *et al*. Recombinant granulocyte-macrophage colony-stimulating factor after autologous bone marrow transplantation for lymphoid cancer. *N Engl J Med* 1991;**324**:1773-8.

Radiotherapy update

A HORWICH

In the narrowest sense radiotherapy is a treatment almost exclusively used in managing cancer and based on the use of ionising radiation. In practice, however, the scope of the subject is broad (box 1) as management decisions relating to cancer must be made in the context of a thorough appraisal of the tumour and patient. Tumours are characterised by histogenesis and morphology, and, increasingly, molecular and genetic analyses are improving the precision and prognostic power of histopathology.[1-3] Assessment of patients must incorporate not only a thorough general medical examination but

---

Box 1 — Functions covered by the specialty of radiotherapy

General medical management of the cancer patient
Clinical and radiological assessments of disease stage
Curative high dose radiotherapy
Palliative radiotherapy
Chemotherapy
Hormone therapy
Biological therapies
Symptom control
Psychological support
Audit
Clinical research
Management
Public education
Teaching and training

Box 2—Clinical roles of radiotherapy

Curative as sole treatment for:
- Head and neck cancers
- Cancer of the cervix
- Seminomas
- Hodgkin's disease and non-Hodgkin's lymphoma
- Bladder cancer
- Early prostate cancer
- Early lung cancer
- Anal and skin cancers
- Medulloblastoma and some other brain tumours
- Thyroid cancer

Component of multimodality curative treatment:
- Breast cancer
- Rectal cancer
- Soft tissue sarcomas
- Advanced head and neck cancers
- Whole body radiotherapy before marrow transplants

Palliative radiotherapy:
- Pain, especially bone metastases
- Bleeding—for example, haemoptysis, haematuria
- Spinal cord compression
- Brain metastases
- Venous or lymphatic obstruction

---

investigation with both established and developing radiological techniques, which can provide sensitive assessments of the extent of disease and may soon be able to give information such as tumour blood flow,[4] cell membrane turnover,[5] proliferative capacity, or degree of oxygenation.[6]

Radiotherapy is used for about half of the 200 000 patients who develop cancer in the United Kingdom each year.[7] It has a curative role in two thirds of patients and a palliative role in the remainder (box 2). Increasingly, management of cancer also involves surgery and chemotherapy.[8] For many cancers the appropriate balance of treatments is still being evaluated, and audit and clinical trials are particularly important in view of the speed and frequency with which treatment advances are brought into clinical practice. Among the problems compounding the difficulties of treating cancer is the need for medical and psychological support for coincidental or treatment related problems and for the anxiety and stress experienced by patients and their relatives at the prospect of a life threatening illness.[9] In the United Kingdom radiotherapists are often also responsible for chemotherapy, and the breadth of management responsibility has led to the renaming of the specialty as clinical oncology.

Clinical role

The role of radiotherapy for particular tumours is determined partly by the average radiosensitivity of the tumour relative to adjacent normal tissues and partly by the probability that the tumour is localised (box 2). Thus radiotherapy has a curative role in cancers of the head and neck; gynaecological tumours, especially carcinoma of the cervix; early lymphomas including Hodgkin's disease; seminoma of the testis; early carcinoma of the prostate; and locally advanced cancers of the bladder. Additionally a small proportion of localised bronchogenic carcinomas can be cured with radiotherapy, and it has a role complementary to surgery in treating breast cancer, rectal cancer, and sarcomas. Improvements in radiotherapy, as with other medical practices, must be judged in terms of therapeutic ratio. Most of the biological effects of radiation are secondary to cytotoxicity and are determined partly by the physical characteristics of the radiation, partly by dose and timing of dose administration (fractionation), and partly by the radiosensitivity of tissue stem cells within the radiation target volume. Knowledge of the radiation sensitivity of the stem cells concerned and accurate anatomical localisation of the treatment are essential to ensure that radiation affects only the tumour.

Recent progress in radiotherapy has derived from three background disciplines—biology, imaging, and radiation physics, especially as applied to linear accelerator technology. The biological basis of the effects of radiation is complex, and the wide range of radiation sensitivity seen in different types of tumour is intriguing.[10] For example, with conventionally fractionated radiotherapy a dose of about 25 Gy is needed to control a 2 cm seminoma, a dose of 35-40 Gy to control a 2 cm lymphoma, and 60-65 Gy an epithelial tumour such as squamous cancer of the head and neck; doses over 70 Gy will not control a similarly sized high grade astrocytoma. Similar ranking of radiosensitivity is seen in the laboratory with cell lines derived from these human tumours.[11]

Determining radiosensitivity

An important goal of current research is to determine the molecular mechanisms underlying differences in radiosensitivity. It seems that there may be differences in induction of damage to DNA, rejoining of DNA strand breaks, or repairing of damaged genes.[12] Analysis of cell lines from patients with ataxia telangiectasia, a recessively inherited syndrome characterised by extreme radiation sensitivity, has been informative.[13] Scientists expect that the gene for the syndrome will be identified and cloned in the near future, which should help to identify at least one mechanism of radiosensitivity. Accurate prediction of individual tumour radiosensitivity is an important research avenue leading to more appropriate and more effective choice of treatment, radiation dose, and fractionation.[14]

At the cellular level it is clear that one mechanism of radiation resistance is rapid proliferation of tumour stem cells during protracted radiotherapy.[15 16] Studies have shown that the potential doubling time of tumour cells is often as short as four days.[17] During a seven week course of radiotherapy this could allow the number of tumour stem cells to increase by a factor of about 10 000. Cellular repopulation of a tumour may be even more efficient after the start of radiotherapy so it is desirable to give radiotherapy as rapidly as possible. Obviously, rapid treatment could be easily managed by giving a large dose of radiotherapy each day; however, this increases the risk of damage to healthy tissue. The solution to this problem has been to give several small doses of radiotherapy per day to shorten the overall treatment time, a strategy known as accelerated fractionation.

Several methods of accelerated fractionation exist, but one of the more extreme is continuous hyperfractioned accelerated radiotherapy (CHART). Pilot studies in non-small cell carcinoma of the bronchus[18] and advanced head and neck cancers[19] gave better results than were achieved in historical controls, and CHART is currently being studied in prospective national trials in Britain.

Improving sensitivity

A second target for improvement of radiotherapy has been based on the observation that tumour tissues have a poorly organised vascular supply and usually contain areas of hypoxic tissue.[20] Laboratory studies show that hypoxia confers resistance to radiation and thus viable but hypoxic tumour cells may be a cause of treatment failure. Hyperbaric oxygen chambers have been used during radiotherapy to improve efficacy,[21] and more recently drugs which mimic the effect of oxygen, such as misonidazole, have also been tried.[22] These drugs were difficult to administer and of only slight benefit. One problem was that misonidazole produced neurotoxicity at high cumulative doses, but the second generation compound etanidazole, which has equivalent sensitising effects in hypoxic tissues, can be given in much higher doses before causing neuropathy[23]; it is currently being investigated in prospective randomised trials in advanced head and neck cancers.

A more recent approach in the United Kingdom which has not yet been evaluated clinically is to use simple oxygen breathing together with nicotinamide, which is thought to improve the tumour's blood supply by inhibiting capillary shut down[24]; animal models suggest that this considerably enhances the effects of radiation and clinical trials are planned.

Chemotherapy

The clinical effects of combining chemotherapy and radiotherapy have been generally disappointing.[25] It would be expected that these treatments, which act by different cellular mechanisms, would be at least additive in effect and, since their side effects tend to be distinct, that additive toxicity would be minimal. In practice the subject is immensely complex because of the variety of chemotherapeutic drugs and drug combinations that could be combined with radiotherapy and the number of different schedules of radiotherapy and chemotherapy, including neoadjuvant chemotherapy, simultaneous chemotherapy, alternating chemotherapy and radiotherapy, or adjuvant chemotherapy after radiotherapy. There has proved to be a considerable risk of enhanced toxicity, especially when drugs and radiation are administered simultaneously.[26]

Clinical experience so far has supported combined chemotherapy and radiotherapy only when each treatment attacks a different target. Examples include systematic control of acute lymphoblastic leukaemia with chemotherapy and irradiation of the chemotherapy sanctuary site within the cerebrospinal fluid space,[27] and early Hodgkin's disease, when a small radiation field is used to treat overt malignant lymphadenopathy and adjuvant chemotherapy to treat the possibility of widespread subclinical disease.[28]

It has proved more difficult to establish a role for combining chemotherapy and radiotherapy to treat the same tumour mass. However, cancer of the anal canal, which is traditionally treated by radical excision and consequent bowel diversion, does seem to be just as successfully treated by relatively low doses of radiotherapy combined with simultaneous 5-fluorouracil and mitomycin C.[29] Even in this example it is as yet unclear whether similar results could be achieved with radiotherapy alone, and this is being compared in a trial by the United Kingdom Coordinating Committee for Cancer Research.

The use of chemotherapy before radiotherapy is thought to offer several advantages. These include a reduction in the amount of tumour to be treated, a reduction in the target volume or amount of normal tissue to be treated, a reduction in the degree of hypoxia in the primary tumour, and the early treatment of subclinical metastatic disease. This approach is currently being evaluated in advanced head and neck cancers, bladder cancer, and advanced cancers of the cervix, among other sites.

New imaging techniques

The second major research pillar of radiotherapy is imaging. The development of computed tomographic scanning arguably had a more profound effect on radiotherapeutic practice than on any other specialty. It has greatly increased the accuracy of tumour staging in respect of the extent of the primary tumour, the presence of local nodal disease in sites relatively difficult to assess such as the mediastinum and abdomen, and the detection of small volume distant metastases. In addition computed tomography enables precise localisation of a tumour or organ within a two dimensional axial slice, the same axis on which radiation treatment plans are designed and calculated.[30] This offers a rapid and accurate computer based system for displaying the effects of alternative radiotherapy isodose plans, usually with combinations of two to four coplanar axial beams and compensating for differential beam attenuation in heterogeneous tissues or by irregular body surface contour.

Computerised planning is now complemented by the development of magnetic resonance imaging (figure). The ability to image directly in the coronal or sagittal plane is of particular benefit and offers greater sensitivity in some sites such as the central nervous system. Sagittal imaging with magnetic resonance imaging has already proved invaluable in diagnosing spinal cord compression. It can be used to define precisely the vertical extent of tumour or normal tissues, thus providing the basis of the development of direct planning of radiotherapy on the magnetic resonance image.

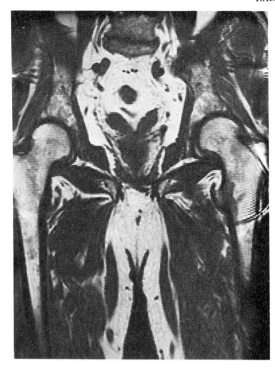

Coronal magnetic resonance imaging showing ability of technique to localise the prostate and seminal vesicles precisely

It is now also possible to produce a three dimensional image by isotopic imaging. Positron emission tomography relies on the use of certain isotope tracers such as fluorine-18, oxygen-15, or iodine-124.[6] The technique can provide both anatomical and functional assessments and has been used, for example, to define precise dosimetry of [124]I in treating iodine avid carcinomas of the thyroid, producing for the first time a rational basis for the dose of isotope and an explanation why certain metastatic sites respond less well to radiation.[31]

Linear accelerator

Developments in the technology of linear accelerator design also offer scope for advances in the precision of radiation treatment. One factor limiting the dose of radiation is the volume of normal tissue within the overall target volume.[32] If the same tumour could be treated and normal tissue excluded then this could either reduce the risk of normal tissue damage or allow escalation of the radiation dose.[33]

117

In the past radiation volumes have usually been cubes of tissue defined by the shape of the aperture of the head of the linear accelerator. The development of precise three dimensional imaging and of computer control of a range of treatment machine parameters now allows much more complex target volumes to be used.[34]. A mechanism for producing these is based on a device called a multileaf collimator. The collimator shapes the edges of the radiation beam and in the past has been a single straight block. The replacement of this single block by a number of independent leaves offers the possibility of treating an irregular shaped tumour while excluding most of the normal tissue. Initial trials are currently quantifying the reduction in toxicity associated with "conformal radiotherapy," and if a reduction can be confirmed the next step will be to investigate dose escalations. Retrospective studies suggest that a dose escalation of 10% would for most tumours improve local control by 10-20%,[35] and the association between local control and survival[36] emphasises the potential of this technique for significantly improving survival from cancer over the next decade.

Future of radiotherapy

Several factors have recently increased the importance of improving cancer therapies. Since cancer is mainly a disease of elderly people the rise in the age distribution of the population will certainly lead to an increased incidence of cancer in the community. At the same time, greater sophistication of surgery and radiotherapy and the development of effective chemotherapy regimens have increased the

---

Box 3—Future developments in radiotherapy

Genetic diagnosis and characterisation
Management of premalignant lesions
Radiosensitising drugs
Isotope immunoconjugates
Conformal radiotherapy and three dimensional planning
Predictive testing of individual tumour and normal tissue
  radiosensitivity
Stem cell manipulation to protect normal tissues
Combined chemotherapy and radiotherapy
Altered radiation fractionation regimens using multiple treatments per
  day

---

complexity of cancer treatments, improving prospects for effective palliation and cure. The rapid pace of research in both cancer biology and technology will ensure exciting advances in the use of radiotherapy in the coming decades (box 3).[37]

1 Brodeur GM, Seeger RC, Varmus HE, Bishop JM. Amplification of N-myc in untreated human neuroblastomas correlates with an advanced disease stage. *Science* 1984;**224**:1121-4.
2 Tandon AK, Clark GM, Chamness GC, Ullrich A, McGuire WL. HER-2/neu oncogene protein and prognosis in breast cancer. *J Clin Oncol* 1989;**7**: 1120-8.
3 Thorpe SM, Rochefort H, Garcia M, Freiss G, Christensen IGJ, Khalaf S, *et al.* Association between high concentrations of M_r 52 000 Cathepsin D and poor prognosis in primary human breast cancer. *Cancer Res* 1989;**49**: 6008-14.
4 Rowell NP, McCready VR, Tait D, Flower MA, Cronin B, Horwich A. Technetium-99m HMPAO and SPECT in the assessment of blood flow in human lung tumours. *Br J Cancer* 1989;**59**:135-41.
5 Glaholm J, Leach MO, Collins DJ, Mansi G, Sharp JC, Madden A, *et al.* In vivo ³¹P magnetic resonance spectroscopy for monitoring treatment response in breast cancer. *Lancet* 1989;i: 1326-7.
6 Ott RJ. The applications of positron emission tomography to oncology. *Br J Cancer* 1991;**63**:343-5.
7 Welsh Office. *Review of the provision of cancer services to the people of north Wales.* Cardiff: Welsh Office, 1989.
8 Rees GJG, Deutsch GP, Dunlop PRC, Priestman TJ. Clinical oncology services to district general hospitals: report of a working party of the Royal College of Radiologists. *Clin Oncol* 1991;**3**:41-5.
9 Moynihan C. Testicular cancer: the psychosocial problem of patients and their relatives. *Cancer Surv* 1987;**5**:477-510.
10 Steel GG, Peacock JH. Why are some human tumours more radiosensitive than others? *Radiother Oncol* 1989;**15**:63-72.
11 Deacon J, Peckham MJ, Steel GG. The radioresponsiveness of human tumours and the initial slope of the cell survival curve. *Radiother Oncol* 1984;**2**:317-24.
12 Powell S, McMillan TJ. DNA damage and repair following treatment with ionizing radiation. *Radiother Oncol* 1990;**19**:95-108.
13 Cox R, Debenham PG, Masson WF, Webb MBT. Ataxia-telangiectasia: a mutation giving a high frequency of misrepair of DNA double-strand scissions. *Mol Biol Med* 1986;**3**:229-44.
14 Parkins C, Horwich A. Prediction of tumour response to treatment. In: Steel GG, Adams GE, Horwich A, eds. *The biological basis of radiotherapy.* 2nd ed. Amsterdam: Elsevier, 1989: 305-17.
15 Withers HR. Biological basis for altered fractionation schemes. *Cancer* 1985;**55**:2086-95.
16 Trott K-R, Kummermehr J. What is known about tumour proliferation rates to choose between accelerated fractionation or hyperfractionation? *Radiother Oncol* 1985;**3**:1-9.
17 Wilson GD, McNally NJ, Dische S, Saundess MI, Des Rochers C, Lewis AA, *et al.* Measurement of cell kinetics in human tumours in vivo using bromodeoxyuridine incorporation and flow cytometry. *Br J Cancer* 1988;**58**: 423-31.
18 Saunders MI, Dische S. Continuous, hyperfractionated, accelerated radiotherapy (CHART) in non-small cell carcinoma of the bronchus. *Int J Radiat Oncol Biol Phys* 1990;**19**:1211-5.
19 Saunders MI, Dische S, Hong A, Grosch EJ, Fermont DC, Ashford RF, *et al.* Continuous hyperfractionated accelerated radiotherapy in locally advanced carcinoma of the head and neck region. *Int J Radiat Oncol Biol Phys* 1989;**17**:1287-93.
20 Thomlinson RH, Gray LH. The histological structure of some human lung cancers and the possible implications for radiotherapy. *Br J Cancer* 1955;**9**:539-49.
21 Henk JM. Does hyperbaric oxygen have a future in radiation therapy? *Int J Radiat Oncol Biol Phys* 1981;**7**:1125-8.
22 Dische S. Chemical sensitizers for hypoxic cells: a decade of experience in clinical radiotherapy. *Radiother Oncol* 1985;**3**:97-115.
23 Coleman CN, Wasserman TH, Urtasun RC, Halsey J, Noll L, Hancock S, *et al.* Final report of the phase I trial of the hypoxic cell radiosensitizer SR-2508 (ethanidazole). Radiation Therapy Oncology Group 83-03. *Int J Radiat Oncol Biol Phys* 1990;**18**:389-93.

24 Chaplin DJ, Olive PL, Durand RE. Intermittent blood flow in a murine tumor: radiobiological effects. *Cancer Res* 1987;**47**:597-601.
25 Horwich A. Combined radiotherapy—chemotherapy in clinical practice. In: Steel GG, Adams GE, Horwich A, eds. *The biological basis of radiotherapy*. Amsterdam: Elsevier, 1989:279-89.
26 Steel GG. The search for therapeutic gain in the combination of radiotherapy and chemotherapy. *Radiother Oncol* 1988;**11**:31-53.
27 Medical Research Council Leukaemia Committee. Treatment of acute lymphoblastic leukaemia: effect of "prophylactic" therapy against central nervous system leukaemia. *BMJ* 1983;ii:381-4.
28 Horwich A, Peckham MJ. Combined chemotherapy and radiotherapy in the management of adult Hodgkin's disease: indications and results. In: Selby P, McElwain TJ, eds. *Hodgkin's disease*. Oxford: Blackwell Scientific, 1987:250-68.
29 Cummings B, Keane TJ, Thomas GM, Harwood AR, Rider WD. Results and toxicity of the treatment of anal canal carcinoma by radiation therapy or radiation therapy and chemotherapy. *Cancer* 1984;**54**:2062-8.
30 Dobbs HJ, Husband JE. Computed tomography for radiotherapy planning. *Appl Radiol* 1984;**13**:51-61.
31 O'Connell MEA, Flower MA, Hinton PJ, Harmer CL, McCread VR. Radioiodine dose assessment. Dose-response in differentiated thyroid carcinoma using quantitative scanning and PET. *Radiother Oncol* (in press).
32 Emami B, Lyman J, Brown A, *et al*. Tolerance of normal tissue to therapeutic irradiation. *Int J Radiat Oncol Biol Phys* 1991;**21**:109-22.
33 Tait D. Conformal therapy. *Br J Cancer* 1990;**62**:702-4.
34 Tait D, Nahum A, Southall C, Chow M, Yarnold JR. Benefits expected from simple conformal radiotherapy in the treatment of pelvic tumours. *Radiother Oncol* 1988;**13**:23-30.
35 Williams MV, Denekamp J, Fowler JF. Dose response relationships for human tumours: implications for clinical trials of dose modifying agents. *Int J Radiat Oncol Biol Phys* 1984;**10**:1703-7.
36 Suit H. Potential for improving survival rates for the cancer patient by increasing the efficacy of treatment of the primary lesion. *Cancer* 1982;**50**: 1227-34.
37 Horwich A. The future of radiotherapy. *Radiother Oncol* 1990;**19**:353-6.

Biological therapy

TIMOTHY PERREN, PETER SELBY

Biological therapy for cancer may be defined as a treatment that uses biological materials, usually cells or cell products, which either have direct effects on tumour cell proliferation or differentiation or modify the host biological response to the malignant disease.[1] The subject has a long history, extending back to the last century, when patients were treated with extracts of infectious organisms or tumours, with occasional success claimed. In the 1970s immunotherapy with BCG and allogeneic or autologous tumour cells was widely investigated, but carefully performed clinical studies failed to show consistent success. However, in the past few years there has been increasing interest in biological therapy for cancer and considerable research activity. In this chapter we will try to explain the reasons for the increasing current interest and discern whether there is really promise of progress.

Potential of biological therapy

The rekindling of interest in biological therapy for cancer followed inevitably from the developments in biology in the 1970s and 1980s. In particular, the techniques and knowledge generated by molecular biologists transformed our understanding of cell proliferation and differentiation and cell to cell interaction in the immune system and elsewhere. The identification of the molecular basis of many biological processes has presented new ideas for biological treatment. Perhaps the best example of this lies in the characterisation of the T cell growth factor interleukin 2, which promotes the proliferation

121

of T lymphocytes as well as stimulates other cytotoxic cell populations and macrophages. The biology of interleukin 2 led to experimental cancer therapy, and Rosenberg *et al* introduced it into the clinic to enhance immune responses against tumours with limited but definite success.[2] In addition, DNA recombinant technology has allowed the expression of the genes for many potent biological materials in prokaryotic or eukaryotic systems, resulting in the production of large quantities that can be readily purified for clinical use. Molecular biology has not only presented the ideas for biological therapies but has also presented us with the means of carrying out those ideas by using recombinant proteins.

Some of the agents now available have direct anticancer effects: interferons have antiproliferative effects; tumour necrosis factors have a direct cytotoxic effect. However, others such as interleukin 2 or interleukin 6 may act by enhancing naturally occurring responses to cancers.[3] Other biological factors may be useful in reducing the toxicity of conventional chemotherapeutic drugs—for example, haemopoietic growth factors ameliorate the bone marrow toxicity of some cytotoxic drugs. The interaction of biological treatments with chemotherapy or radiotherapy offers valuable combined approaches which already have shown some promise.[4]

Although current interest has concentrated on recombinant proteins, other biological approaches including monoclonal antibodies, active immunisation, and adoptive cellular therapy are being studied. Monoclonal antibodies directed against tumour associated antigens have been used as anticancer agents in many centres and tumour regression has been described, although it is uncommon and short lived so far. Antibodies to idiotypic immunoglobulin determinants on B lymphomas are a theoretically attractive treatment because each idiotype is tumour specific, but results are still disappointing, as are those for monoclonal antibodies to antigens associated with melanoma and epithelial cancers. Improvements may come from clearer understanding of basic immunology, genetically engineered antibodies, or the use of monoclonal antibodies in combination treatments.[5 6] Active immunisation with melanoma tumour antigens can apparently produce tumour regression[7] and needs further research. Adoptive transfer of cells achieved popularity after the work of Rosenberg *et al*[2] but has not been proved to add to the effects of interleukin 2.[8]

Cytokines

The recombinant proteins of greatest current interest are cytokines. Cytokines are low molecular weight polypeptides (usually less than 80 kDa) produced by a wide range of cell types. They usually act locally in a paracrine or autocrine fashion but may remain bound to the cell surface in some circumstances. They are produced in response to inducing signals, have a short half life and high biological potency, bind to high affinity specific cell surface receptors, and affect cellular growth (stimulation or inhibition) or cellular differentiation, or both.[19] Cytokines have usually been discovered as the result of the identification of a particular action, such as the antiviral effect of interferons or the T cell growth effects of interleukin 2. They almost all have multiple actions, and the first activity described may not be the most important to the oncologist. The table lists the cytokines which are being clinically evaluated or are nearing clinical trials, together with known actions and therapeutic potential. The list is impressive, the biology complex, and the therapeutic potential considerable. There are a few common themes about our present state of evaluation of cytokine therapy.

Firstly, several cytokines have definite anticancer activity in humans. Interferon alfa, interferon gamma, and interleukin 2 have a small but consistent effect against haemopoietic cancers, renal cancer, and melanoma and less consistent effects against other cancers.[5] The activity of tumour necrosis factor is much less, and the value of interleukin 4, interleukin 6, and the growth factors or their antagonists is much less clear. Secondly, so far (with the exception of interferon against hairy cell leukaemia) the effects are small and benefits are found in a minority of patients.

Thirdly, we still do not know how to use any cytokine properly. The ideal dose and schedule of interferon alfa has not been established precisely despite 15 years of clinical research, and the optimal dose, schedule, and route of administration for interleukin 2 are still unknown. Most studies have aimed at finding a use for cytokines in treating established, advanced, and poor prognosis cancers. There is some evidence suggesting that their most useful role is as a maintenance treatment given after initial induction of remission by chemotherapy, surgery, or radiotherapy.

Lastly, cytokines have so far been quite toxic.[139] The pleotrophic effects on cells and organisms seen in the laboratory are manifest as adverse reactions when cytokines are used in the clinic. Febrile

Action and therapeutic effects of cytokines

Name	Action	Therapeutic effects
Interferon alfa	Antiviral, antiproliferative, immunomodulatory	Remissions in renal cancer, melanoma, hairy cell leukaemia, and chronic leukaemia. Maintenance in myeloma
Interferon gamma	Activation of natural killer cells and macrophages	Some antitumour activity
Granulocyte colony stimulating factor Macrophage colony stimulating factor Granulocyte macrophage colony stimulating factor Interleukin 3	Stimulation of haemopoietic progenitor cells in bone marrow to proliferate and differentiate producing colonies of mature end cells. Enhancement of end cell function. Granulocyte and macrophage factors are lineage restricted, granulocyte macrophage factor and interleukin 3 affect all three lineages	Enhancement of bone marrow recovery and end cell function. Increased dose and frequency of chemotherapy. Reduction in incidence of, and faster recovery from, infection
Interleukin 2	Expansion and activation of T (and B) lymphocytes	Antitumour agent in renal cancer and melanoma
Interleukin 4	B cell growth factor, increase T cytotoxicity, inhibit lymphokine activated killer cell formation	Early clinical trials
Interleukin 6	B cell growth factor. Modulates haemopoietic progenitor cells to respond to lineage restricted factors	Use of antagonists or antibodies in myeloma and autoimmune disease. Anticancer effect in laboratory
Tumour necrosis factor	Cytotoxicity in vitro and model systems	Occasional antitumour activity. Antibodies to tumour necrosis factor may lessen severity of shock
Epidermal growth factor Transforming growth factor alfa Platelet derived growth factor Transforming growth factor β	Fibroblast growth stimulation Growth inhibition Growth stimulation or inhibition depending on cell concerned and the presence of other factors	Overproduction of the factors or abnormal expression of their receptors, or both, may stimulate proliferation of malignant cells. Molecular variants of factors or role receptors have putative role as anticancer agents

reactions, endothelial toxicity, hypotension, and renal toxicity have all been seen. The toxicities are different from those associated with conventional cytotoxic chemotherapy but are not less severe. The reagents have to be handled with the greatest care in the clinic.

Clinical activity of cytokines

Interferons

Interferon alfa, for which there are at least 20 genes on chromosome 9, is in many ways the prototype cytokine. Interferons beta and gamma are encoded by single genes on chromosomes 9 and 12 and a distinct role for them has not yet been determined despite some biological differences from interferon alfa.[10]

Interferon extracted from leucocytes was introduced into clinical practice in the 1970s and the initial effects were promising, particularly in the treatment of multiple myeloma and osteosarcoma. Unfortunately, this promise was not sustained when larger numbers of patients were treated and interferon fell largely into disrepute. This situation has been altered as a result of five observations:

• A large and consistent benefit for patients with hairy cell leukaemia, a rare form of leukaemia mainly in middle aged men, was observed.[11] Although not curative, giving interferon alfa transformed the prognosis of patients with this disease with clinical remissions and excellent quality of life after the introduction of treatment.

• Responses to interferon with reduction in tumour volume were seen with several relatively common solid cancers such as renal cancer, melanoma, and neuroendocrine tumours. These effects occurred in a substantial minority of patients but were not usually longlasting and probably never curative.[3]

• Interferon alfa is capable of maintaining remissions induced by chemotherapy, especially in multiple myeloma and non-Hodgkin's lymphoma, despite its rather poor performance in treating patients who have active or advanced diseases.[12] Very few other anticancer treatments can maintain remissions. Even diseases like Hodgkin's disease or testicular cancer which are very sensitive to cytotoxic chemotherapy do not benefit from prolonged maintenance chemotherapy. The discovery of any treatment that can maintain remissions, particularly when these remissions are relatively frequent, as in the haemopoietic cancers, must be welcomed and explored further. Interferon alfa may be particularly important in epithelial cancers such as breast and ovarian cancers in which responses to chemotherapy occur in most patients with advanced disease but most die as a result of relapses within one or two years.

• Interferon alfa combined with cytotoxic chemotherapy seems to increase the response rate significantly, with lengthy remissions extending to one or two years reported in some patients with advanced colorectal cancer.[4] Although not yet confirmed by a randomised prospective trial, this treatment seems to offer the prospect of useful remissions in this drug resistant disease.

• Prolonged treatment with interferon alfa seems to be capable of producing cytogenetically defined remissions of chronic granulocytic leukaemia.[13]

Interleukin 2

The scientific basis of treatment with interleukin 2 was among the most exciting topics in oncology in the 1980s. The prospect of an agent that directly amplifies immune responses to tumours was greeted with great enthusiasm. Rosenberg et al showed that high doses of interleukin 2 given together with the passive transfer of lymphocytes which had been stimulated by interleukin 2 in vitro were capable of producing remissions in a substantial minority of patients with a wide range of cancers, particularly renal cancer and melanoma.[7] However, there was high associated toxicity. More recent work using different methods of administration, such as continuous intravenous infusion or subcutaneous injections, has confirmed that this approach is capable of producing tumour regressions and that some of these remissions last several years, with some evidence of prolonged survival (M Jones et al, unpublished data).

Tumour necrosis factor

In many ways tumour necrosis factor has been the most disappointing of the cytokines tried as potential cancer treatments.[14] It is the only cytokine whose existence was suspected as the result of the discovery of anticancer activity in the serum of mice primed with BCG and then exposed to endotoxins. It exerts powerful antitumour effects in model systems both directly on cells in vitro and indirectly in vivo, probably through its effects on endothelial cells and the resulting destruction of tumour vasculature. Secondary release of other cytokines may also be important in the effects of tumour necrosis factor. In humans, however, it is toxic and associated with only occasional regressions of cancer,[14] and the concentrations achievable in the

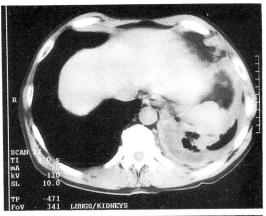

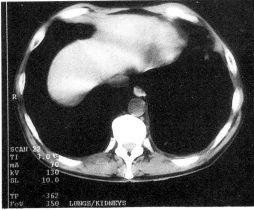

Scan of patient with metastatic renal carcinoma with pleural and pulmonary disease (top) and hypercalcaemia. Treatment with 20 day intravenous interleukin 2 cleared his disease, except for small area of pleural thickening (bottom). Remission continued at 6 months

blood of patients are much lower than those which are necessary to produce regressions of cancers in experimental models.[1 14] Better understanding of the biology of tumour necrosis factor, its inhibitors, and its interaction with other cytokines and with cytotoxic drugs may yet find it a useful role as an anticancer drug. At present such a use is highly speculative, and in some circumstances tumour necrosis factor can stimulate tumour growth in vitro.

Haemopoietic growth factors

The evidence that haemopoietic growth factors can stimulate the bone marrow in humans and reduce myelosuppression by cytotoxic drugs is now conclusive.[15-17] These agents have an established role in treating patients with life threatening sepsis with neutropenia. The

127

lineage specificity of the available haemopoietic growth factors means that their value is greatest for patients with neutropenia. Whether the marrow stimulation achieved with haemopoietic growth factors will result in a general improvement in prognosis for patients with cancer is unclear. Sepsis is reduced, but most neutropenic sepsis can be handled safely with modern antibiotics. Perhaps the central question is whether haemopoietic growth factors will allow increased doses of cytotoxic drugs and whether this will result in more remissions and perhaps more cures. Although increased tolerance to chemotherapy can be achieved, it is not yet clear that the dose escalation which is possible will result in major benefits in terms of quantity or quality of life for patients.[17]

Conclusion

Biological treatments, particularly DNA recombinant cytokines, have an established place in the management of some human cancers. Induction of long term remission in hairy cell leukaemia by interferon, maintenance of remission in multiple myeloma, and the treatment of renal cancer with interferon or interleukin 2 are now part of established practice in oncology in many centres and are recognised by regulatory authorities in most European countries. The mechanisms of action of cytokines clearly present possibilities different from those of cytotoxic chemotherapy. However, the benefits of biological therapies at present are relatively small and limited to a small proportion of patients.

It is too early to conclude that further research into biological therapy will result in larger benefits for larger numbers of such patients. There are, however, some encouraging signs. In 1992 biological therapy is in a position rather similar to that of chemotherapy in the 1940s. A small number of active reagents exist, only a minority of patients with any particular disease seem to respond, and the responses are usually of short duration with occasional durable remissions or cures. In the three decades after the 1940s chemotherapy developed rapidly, with new drugs, combination chemotherapy, high dose treatments, and adjuvant chemotherapy. These led to impressive advances in treatment of paediatric cancers, haemopoietic cancers, and germ cell tumours, resulting in the cure of many patients with these cancers by the early 1980s. Will the next few decades see similar advances in our understanding and use of biological therapy? Will these advances occur this time in common cancers? The evidence available certainly suggests that research into this application of the new biology to medicine is worth pursuing.

TP and PS are supported by the Yorkshire Cancer Research Campaign.

1 Jones A, Selby P. Biological therapies. *Radiother Oncol* 1991;**20**:211-23.
2 Rosenberg SA, Aebersold P, Cornetta K, Kasid A, Morgan RA, Moen R. Gene transfer into humans—immunotherapy of melanoma using tumour-infiltrating lymphocytes modified by retroviral gene transduction. *N Engl J Med* 1990;**323**:570-3.
3 De Vita V, Hellman S, Rosenberg SA, eds. *Biologic therapy of cancer*. Philadelphia: J B Lippincott, 1991.
4 Wadler S, Lambersky B, Atkins M, Kirkwood J, Petrelli N. Phase II trial of fluorouracil and recombinant interferon alfa-2a in patients with advanced colorectal carcinoma. An Eastern Cooperative Oncology Group study. *J Clin Oncol* 1991;**9**:1806-10.
5 Hale G, Clark MR, Marcus R. Remission induction in non-Hodgkin lymphoma with re-shaped human monoclonal antibody CAMPATH-1H. *Lancet* 1988;**ii**:1394-9.
6 Honsik CJ, Jung G, Reisfeld RA. Lymphokine-activated killer cells targeted by monoclonal antibodies to the disialogangliosides GD2 and GD3 specifically lyse human tumour cells of neuroectodermal origin. *Proc Nat Acad Sci USA* 1986;**83**:7893-7.
7 Mitchell MS, Kan-Mitchell J, Kempf RA, Harel W, Shau HY, Lind S. Active specific immunotherapy for melanoma: phase I trial of allogeneic lysates and a novel adjuvant. *Cancer Res* 1988;**48**:5883.
8 Palmer PA, Vinke J, Evers P. A review of patients treated by continuous infusion of recombinant interleukin-2 (rIL-2) with or without autologous lymphokine activated killer cells for the treatment of advanced renal cell carcinoma. *Eur J Cancer* (in press).
9 Balkwill F, Burke F. The cytokine network. *Immunology Today* 1989;**10**:299-303.
10 Kurzrock R, Gutterman JU, Talpay M. Interferons alfa, beta and gamma; basic principles and pre-clinical studies. In: De Vita V, Hellman S, Rosenberg SA, eds. *Biologic Therapy of Cancer*. Philadelphia: J B Lippincott, 1991:247-74.
11 Quesada JR, Itri L, Gutterman JU. Alfa interferon in hairy cell leukaemia: a five year follow up in 100 patients. *Journal of International Research* 1988;**6**:678-85.
12 Mandelli F, Avvisati G, Amadori S, Boccadoro M, Genong A, Lauta VM. Maintenance treatment with alfa-2b recombinant interferon significantly improves response and survival duration in multiple myeloma patients responding to conventional induction chemotherapy. Results of an Italian randomised study. *N Engl J Med* 1990;**322**:1430-4.
13 Talpaz M, Kantarjian HM, McCredie KB, Trijillo JM, Keating MJ, Guttermang JW. Hematologic remission and cytogenetic improvement induced by recombinant human interferon alfa in chronic myelogenous leukaemia. *N Engl J Med* 1986;**314**:1065.
14 Jones AL, Selby P. Tumour necrosis factor: clinical relevance. *Cancer Surv* 1989;**8**:817-36.
15 Crawford J, Ozer H, Stoller R, Johnson D, Lyman G, Tabbara I. Reduction by granulocyte colony-stimulating factor of fever and neutropenia induced by chemotherapy in patients with small cell lung cancer. *N Engl J Med* 1991;**325**:164-70.
16 Scarffe JH. Emerging clinical uses for GM-CSF. *Eur J Cancer* 1991;**27**:1493-504.
17 Ohno R, Tomonaga M, Kobayashi T, Kanamaru A, Shirakawa S, Masauka T. Effect of granulocyte colony-stimulating factor after intensive induction therapy in relapsed or refractory acute leukemia. *N Engl J Med* 1990;**323**:1871-77.

Quality of life: philosophical question or clinical reality?

MAURICE L SLEVIN

Quality of life is the new catch phrase in cancer medicine. Like happiness it is one of those terms that we all understand but for which adequate definitions do not exist. The focus on quality of life for cancer patients has come with the realisation that while dramatic improvements have taken place in the treatment of the less common cancers, and while adjuvant chemotherapy has improved the cure rate for several common cancers when diagnosed and treated in the early stages, most advanced common cancers remain incurable. In these circumstances treatment is given with the intention of providing maximum prolongation of good quality life. This, however, is not always a simple task as the treatment required for the cancer is often associated with side effects which can impair quality of life.

Cancer and its treatment often create havoc and chaos in the lives of patients and their families while other diseases such as ischaemic heart disease, which are a greater cause of death in the population, do not invoke the same degree of panic. Patients with metastatic cancer often have only minor symptoms and have to cope with the realisation that something has been growing inside them without their knowledge and while they were feeling well. This lack of symptoms may paradoxically make the illness seem more frightening and less controllable. In addition, the cause of the illness cannot usually be explained, the description of the disease is likely to be complex and confusing, and it is apparent that even the experts do not have all the answers. Furthermore, people are often told "there is nothing we can do for you," and this error is often compounded by an inaccurate prediction such as "you have six months or a year to live." It is therefore not surprising that patients with cancer often feel more miserable and despondent than patients with other potentially fatal illnesses and that quality of life is a much bigger issue in cancer than it is in other equally life threatening diseases.

It is now generally agreed that quality of life should be measured as an integral component of most cancer trials, particularly where treatments are given with palliative intent.[1] However, this is easier said than done. Time is short in busy cancer clinics, and with increasing emphasis on trials including large numbers of patients carried out mainly in district general hospitals the logistics are formidable.

In practice quality of life data can usually be collected in only a subset of patients within a trial and particularly in those centres where specialist nurses are available. Provided randomisation takes place within each centre this should not introduce significant bias.

Which instruments should we use?

A vast array of quality of life questionnaires is currently on offer. Maguire and Selby carried out an excellent review of available measures on behalf of the Medical Research Council Cancer Therapy Committee.[2] They assessed several instruments looking at clinical utility, ease of administration, and scoring and also reliability and validity. They concluded that the best current method for assessing the key dimensions of quality of life was the Rotterdam symptom checklist.[3] The hospital anxiety depression scale[4] was also particularly useful for assessing anxiety and depression.

The Rotterdam symptom checklist comprises 30 items, each rated on a 4 point scale measuring physical and psychological dimensions of quality of life. It is easy to score and can be divided into different subsets. There are two main subscales, one for physical complaints and one for psychological issues. It has been suggested that this scale does not adequately cover sexual or social dimensions of quality of life and additional physical items have been proposed for use with specific groups of cancer patients.

The hospital anxiety and depression scale was specifically designed to measure anxiety and depression in patients who were physically ill and therefore excluded somatic symptoms of depression, such as weight loss and constipation, which might also be related to the illness. It is a self rating scale and has two subscales for anxiety and depression. Its validity has been confirmed in several studies. It has the advantage of being short and easy to understand and having a simple scoring system. A score of 7 or less implies normality, 8 or 10 is borderline, and 11 or more suggests significant anxiety or depression.

These two scales thus represent the most practical and reliable measures for assessing the quality of life at this time. The European Organisation for Research and Treatment in Cancer questionnaire,[5] which is currently in the final stages of development and validation, offers the possibility of a scale which is easy to score and is designed to measure key dimensions including symptoms of disease, side effects of treatments, physical functioning, psychological distress, social interaction, sexuality, body image, and satisfaction of medical care. This scale will also have modules to make it specifically applicable to individual cancers.

The questions of validity and reliability should be left to the appropriate experts. What is clear is that any form that takes more than a few minutes to fill out will in practice not be completed on a regular basis, and any questionnaire which is difficult to score will not prove feasible. The questionnaires must also be completed by the patients as doctors and nurses are notoriously unreliable at estimating patients' quality of life. assessments on the same patients vary greatly among different doctors and nurses.[6]

The incorporation of quality of life measures in clinical studies is fortunately receiving a higher priority and often provides information which would be unobtainable by other means. The overall balance of benefit versus toxicity, especially where the treatment is given with palliative intent, can be obtained only by careful documentation of quality of life. Despite the limitations of the current instruments their use has already provided fascinating and often non-intuitive information in clinical trials.

Surgical patients

An evaluation of quality of life and functional results after surgery for gastric cancer showed clear evidence of the superiority of total gastrectomy or distal gastrectomy over proximal gastric resection.[7] This goes against the conventional wisdom that total gastrectomy is associated with greater morbidity than partial gastrectomy, which has meant that total gastrectomy was often not used despite its advantages in achieving adequate safety margins. As a result of this trial the authors concluded that proximal gastric resection gave inferior quality of life to total gastrectomy and the last technique should therefore be preferred.

Several studies have compared quality of life after mastectomy with that after breast conserving treatment for carcinoma of the breast. A review of these studies found no solid proof of more favourable psychological adjustment after breast conserving treatment, indicating that these women need as much counselling support as patients who have mastectomy.[8] However, several studies reported better body image and sexual functioning after breast conserving treatment.[9-12] The assumed disadvantage of breast conserving treatment, that women would experience a greater fear of recurrence, was not evident in these studies. In fact, this fear seemed more intense after mastectomy. These studies have been extremely helpful in enabling doctors to guide patients as to the likely psychological effects of either procedure and to focus support where it is most needed.

Chemotherapy: striking a balance

Quality of life evaluations have similarly helped our understanding of the effect of chemotherapy on patients' lives. A particularly difficult subject is the use of adjuvant chemotherapy in premenopausal patients with breast cancer. The problem with adjuvant therapy is that all patients are exposed to significant side effects for benefit in only a proportion of the patients.

A recent study looked at a large randomised trial comparing a single cycle of preoperative adjuvant chemotherapy with six cycles of conventionally timed chemotherapy.[13] The quality of life would be expected to be significantly worse with the longer, more intensive chemotherapy but at five year follow up the patients who had received the longer therapy had better five year survival than those who received a single preoperative cycle. The quality of life was evaluated by using Q-twist, which looks at the quality adjusted time without symptoms. Despite the greater initial toxicity with the more intensive and longer chemotherapy these patients had a longer freedom from disease and less time with the problems of recurrent disease and its treatment. There was thus an improvement in both quantity and quality of life for patients who received the more intensive therapy. With longer follow up this difference would be likely to increase.

One of the earliest studies looking at the effect of treatment on quality of life in advanced breast cancer was carried out by Priestman and Baum in the mid-1970s.[14] This study used linear analogue self assessment scales to compare subjective responses in a trial of patients with advanced breast cancer randomised to endocrine or cytotoxic treatment. The higher response rate in patients receiving cytotoxic chemotherapy correlated with a better overall quality of life than that found in patients receiving endocrine therapy despite the higher incidence of side effects with cytotoxic chemotherapy.

Another trial in advanced breast cancer was conducted by the Australian/New Zealand breast cancer trial group, which randomised patients to receive either continuous or intermittent combination chemotherapy.[15] In the patients receiving intermittent therapy treatment was stopped after three cycles if the disease did not progress. If the disease later progressed the treatment was given for a further three cycles. The other arm of the study received continuous chemotherapy. The results of this study were counterintuitive. Overall quality of life, response to treatment, and time to ultimate treatment failure all favoured continuous therapy. One possible explanation is that patients who were receiving intermittent chemotherapy had increased anxiety when they were not having treatment. However, the changes in quality of life were also found to be significant independent predictors of survival. This suggested that the quality of life reflected the state of the metastatic disease and that the increased side effects of chemotherapy were outweighed by the benefit the patients received from having better disease control.

In the early 1980s Gough et al looked at quality of life in a group of patients with advanced colorectal cancer who were treated with chemotherapy of relatively low toxicity.[16] Although only a few

---

Chemotherapy and quality of life

- More effective therapy is usually associated with better quality of life
- More intensive treatment is therefore not always associated with lower quality of life
- Side effects may be less important than control of disease
- Patients may report improved quality of life despite showing no objective response. This could be related to
  - minimal tumour shrinkage, giving relief of symptoms
  - increased medical attention
  - provision of hope

patients achieved an objective response, most felt that they had benefited from chemotherapy. Several possible reasons for this benefit can be suggested, including placebo effect, provision of hope, or increased medical attention associated with being in a study.

A Scandinavian study looking at two regimens of chemotherapy in advanced symptomatic colorectal cancer provides further insight into the relation between disease control and quality of life.[17] Only a few patients with advanced colorectal cancer respond and chemotherapy is given with palliative intent. The negative effect of chemotherapy on the majority of patients who did not respond might be expected to lead to an overall reduction in quality of life. In this study 22 patients were randomised to single agent 5-fluorouracil and 22 to 5-fluorouracil combined with methotrexate and leucovorin rescue. The response rate was greater with the more intensive chemotherapy. With the 5-fluorouracil alone one patient had a partial response and two had stable disease, whereas with the more intensive chemotherapy five had partial remissions and seven had prolonged stationary disease. The more intensive therapy was, however, also associated with more side effects. Despite the increased side effects 55% of patients given combined chemotherapy rated themselves as having improved quality of life compared with only 9% of the single agent group. The side effects of treatment influenced quality of life ratings negatively in only one patient. This suggests that the intensive chemotherapy was superior as palliative treatment in this study.

Advanced non-small cell lung cancer is particularly difficult to treat, being only moderately radiosensitive, and intensive chemotherapy including cisplatin gives a response in only 20-40% of patients with very minor effects on survival. A Norwegian study compared the quality of life in patients with non-small cell lung cancer randomised to receive either radiotherapy or chemotherapy.[18] Quality of life decreased in the chemotherapy treated patients two weeks after starting treatment. However, after this there was a general improvement in the quality of life for both the chemotherapy and the radiotherapy groups despite the fact that the chemotherapy was repeated every third week for four cycles and that treatment related side effects did not decrease during the second, third, and fourth cycles of chemotherapy. This study again suggests that side effects were not the major determinants of quality of life. The overall improvement in quality of life in both groups, despite a response in only a minority, suggests that the benefits may be related to the optimism and support provided by close medical supervision.

Alternative medicine

Many patients with advanced cancers that are incurable with conventional treatment seek alternative methods of treatment. Practitioners of alternative medicine claim that the non-toxic natural therapies may result in cures and prolongation of life and undoubtedly give a better quality of life. A study from the United States compared a group of patients with advanced cancer treated by a conventional oncologist in a standard medical setting with a carefully matched group who were receiving conventional treatment as well as alternative therapy at a well known clinic.[19] The alternative regimen included injections of BCG and a vaccine said to enhance the patients' natural immunity as well as a strict vegetarian diet and coffee enemas. The study was not randomised as patients who received the alternative therapy were self selecting. This is clearly a limitation of this study. The study found no difference in survival between the two groups but the quality of life scores were consistently better among patients treated with conventional therapy, despite the fact that a greater proportion of these patients had received chemotherapy with the attendant side effects. The patients who had selected themselves to receive alternative therapy may have had unknown factors which contributed to their poorer quality of life, but the study suggests that the assumption that alternative therapies necessarily enhance the quality of life is not valid.

It is clear from these studies that many factors contribute towards quality of life in patients with cancer, including quality of symptom control. Symptom control may be related to the effectiveness of therapy, social functioning, the degree of emotional support, and the extent to which the patient feels hopeful and optimistic. Maximum symptom control is the first priority in trying to improve quality of life. It is a nonsense to focus on emotional support when someone has uncontrollable pain or vomiting. One of the main arguments in favour of patients with advanced incurable cancer seeing cancer specialists is the availability of expertise in symptom control which may be lacking in non-specialist centres. It is also clear from the above quality of life studies that the control of the disease may be an important aspect of symptom control even when the effect of treatment on survival is minimal.

Cost versus benefit in cancer treatment

The provision of hope is one aspect that is rarely addressed by

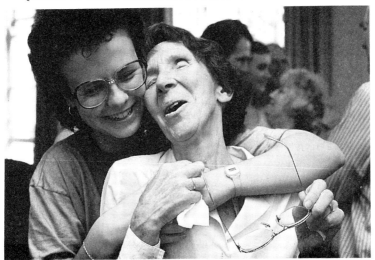

Good palliative treatment and counselling help improve quality of life

doctors, being more in the realm of philosophers than of the medical profession. However, a study asking patients with cancer, about to undergo chemotherapy, to balance the price they were prepared to pay in terms of side effects for a particular degree of benefit showed that most patients would accept toxic chemotherapy for minimal benefit in terms of survival or prolongation of life.[20] This result was not changed when the patients were given the questionnaire after receiving chemotherapy. This shows the extent to which many people require hope at almost any price. This is not an excuse for giving inappropriate toxic and expensive therapy to patients with little or no chance of benefit. However, it does emphasise that a part of the benefit patients obtain from palliative chemotherapy is the hope that treatment brings. It explains why patients enter trials of experimental therapy despite being told that the chances of benefit are small.

Similar results were found in a study looking at what improvement in survival would justify six months of adjuvant chemotherapy for breast cancer. Women who had received adjuvant chemotherapy were asked what improvement in survival would make such treatment worth while. Almost half of the women judged that a 1% improvement in five year survival would justify treatment. A 10% improvement in five year survival would be acceptable to 80% of the women who were treated. These women had all received cytotoxic adjuvant

137

chemotherapy for their breast cancer and were therefore in a good position to evaluate the toxicity of treatment.

Emotional support

Emotional support is something which doctors may feel is more appropriately delegated to nurses, psychologists, or social workers. However, a study asking cancer patients from whom they most wanted and most got emotional support showed that their first choice was their doctor and that the more senior doctors were seen as being capable of giving more emotional support.[21] Undoubtedly patients have much less time with the senior doctors than with more junior doctors and nurses and these data are therefore somewhat paradoxical. It must be concluded that patients get emotional support from receiving what they believe to be accurate and authoritative information. This is probably the single most important means of overcoming panic and restoring a sense of control over a patient's life. However, information is not always positive and the quality of delivery of information may be important.[22] It is almost always negative to tell people that they have a fixed life expectancy. The averages apply to populations and not to individuals and to give people a fixed life expectancy removes hope and provokes depression and despondency. It is more appropriate and helpful to indicate that while life might be very short if things go badly, the length of life could still be long and cannot be estimated if things go well.[23]

Counselling patients with cancer

There is considerable evidence that counselling patients with cancer is helpful in relieving anxiety and depression and in improving fighting spirit and quality of life. Counselling need not be prolonged and indefinite as a recent study of adjuvant psychological therapy, using an average of six hours of counselling, has shown.[24] There is even a suggestion (as yet unconfirmed) from a randomised trial that group therapy for patients with cancer may improve survival.[25]

Many patients with cancer undoubtedly experience severe psychological distress. Despite this the proportion of patients with cancer who accept counselling, even when it is available, remains low. Counselling is a routine part of the management of patients with HIV related diseases and it seems a pity that it is not incorporated as part of the standard package of treatment offered to patients with advanced cancer, especially those being treated with palliative intent.

Conclusions

Today we are in a better position to treat patients with palliative chemotherapy with minimisation of side effects than ever before. The use of effective modern single agents for palliative chemotherapy, which cause less side effects, together with symptom control with drugs such as ondansetron or granisetron, which reduce nausea and vomiting, allows doctors to offer patients a chance of benefit with minimal cost and maintain a hopeful outlook. Quality of life studies comparing modern single agent therapy with combination chemotherapy in advanced cancers are now needed.

Research into quality of life cannot compete for the spotlight with treatment designed to improve survival, and indeed it would be inappropriate for it to do so. However, the current reality is that most advanced cancers are treated with palliative intent and quality of life issues are of primary concern. The quality of symptom control, the use of the least toxic effective chemotherapy, possibly going back to single agents in many cases, may significantly reduce the physical effects of cancer and its treatment. In addition doctors can contribute substantially to emotional support by understanding the patient's need for information, thereby giving them back a sense of control while not removing all hope.

1 Brinkley D. Quality of life in cancer trials. *BMJ* 1985;**291**:685-6.
2 Maguire P, Selby P. Assessing quality of life in cancer patients. *Br J Cancer* 1989;**60**:437-40.
3 de Haes JCJM, van Knippenberg FCE, Neijt JP. Measuring psychological and physical distress in cancer patients: structure and application of the Rotterdam symptom checklist. *Br J Cancer* 1990;**62**:1034-8.
4 Zigmond AS, Snaith RP. The hospital anxiety and depression scale. *Acta Psychiatr Scand* 1983;**67**:361.
5 Aaronson NK, Bullinger M, Ahmedzai S. A modular approach to quality of life assessment in cancer clinical trials. *Recent Results Cancer Res* 1988;**111**:231-49.
6 Slevin ML, Plant H, Lynch D, Drinkwater J, Gregory WM. Who should measure the quality of life, the doctor or the patient? *Br J Cancer* 1988;**57**:109-12.
7 Buhl K, Schlag P, Herfarth C. Quality of life and functional results following different types of resection for gastric carcinoma. *Eur J Surg Oncol* 1990;**16**:404-9.
8 Kiebert GM, de Haes JCJM, van de Velde CJH. The impact of breast-conserving treatment and mastectomy on the quality of life of early-stage breast cancer patients: a review. *J Clin Oncol* 1991;**9**:1059-70.
9 Beckmann J, Johansen L, Richardt C, Blichert-Toft M. Psychological reactions in younger women operated on for breast cancer. *Dan Med Bull* 1983;**30**(suppl 2):10-3.
10 Steinberg MD, Juliano MA, Wise L. Psychological outcome of lumpectomy versus mastectomy in the treatment of breast cancer. *Am J Psychiatry* 1985;**142**:34-9.

11 Taylor SE, Lichtman RR, Wood JV, Bluming AZ, Dosik GM, Leibowitz RL. Illness-related and treatment-related factors in psychosocial adjustment to breast cancer. *Cancer* 1985;55: 2506-13.

12 Wolberg WH, Romsaas EP, Tanne MA, Malec JS. Psychosexual adaptation to breast cancer surgery. *Cancer* 1989;63:1645-55.

13 Gelber RD, Goldhirsch A, Cavalli F. Quality-of-life-adjusted evaluation of adjuvant therapies for operable breast cancer. *Ann Intern Med* 1991;114:621-8.

14 Priestman T, Baum M. Evaluation of quality of life in patients receiving treatment for advanced breast cancer. *Lancet* 1976;i:899-901.

15 Coates A, Gebski V, Bishop J, Jeal PN, Woods RL, Snyder R, *et al*. Improving the quality of life during chemotherapy for advanced breast cancer. A comparison of intermittent and continuous treatment strategies. *N Engl J Med* 1987;317:1490-5.

16 Gough IR, Furnival GM, Burnett W. Patient attitudes to chemotherapy for advanced gastrointestinal cancer. *Clin Oncol* 1981;7:5-11.

17 Glimelius B, Hoffman K, Olafsdottir M, Pahlman L, Sjoden P, Wennberg A. Quality of life during cytostatic therapy for advanced symptomatic colorectal carcinoma: a randomized comparison of two regimens. *Eur J Cancer Clin Oncol* 1989;25:829-35.

18 Kaasa S, Mastekaasa A, Naess S. Quality of life of lung cancer patients in a randomized clinical trial evaluated by a psychosocial well-being questionnaire. *Acta Oncologica* 1988;27:335-42.

19 Cassileth BR, Lusk EJ, DuPont G, Blake A, Walsh WP, Lauren K, *et al*. Survival and quality of life among patients receiving unproven as compared with conventional cancer therapy. *N Engl J Med* 1991;324:1180-5.

20 Slevin ML, Stubbs L, Plant HJ, Wilson P, Gregory WM, Armes PJ, *et al*. Attitudes to chemotherapy: comparing views of patients with cancer with those of doctors, nurses, and general public. *BMJ* 1990;300:1458-60.

21 Slevin ML, Downer S, Cody M, Maher J, Arnott S, Godlee N, *et al*. The evaluation of emotional support by patients with cancer. *Br J Cancer* 1991;63:11.

22 Maguire P, Faulkner A. How to communicate with cancer patients: handling bad news and difficult questions. *BMJ* 1988;297:907-9.

23 Harris J. *The value of life—an introduction to medical ethics*. London: Routledge and Kegan Paul, 1985:87-110.

24 Greer S, Moorey S, Baruch J, Watson M, Robertson B, Mason A, *et al*. Adjuvant psychological therapy for patients with cancer: a prospective randomised trial. *BMJ* 1992;304:675-80.

25 Spiegel D, Bloom JR, Kraemer HC, Gottheil E. Effect of psychosocial treatment on survival of patients with metastatic breast cancer. *Lancet* 1989;ii:888-91.

Index